ALLE ZEIT WACH
1842
SP

Ovarian Cancer

Edited by Norman M. Bleehen

With 48 Figures and 46 Tables

Springer-Verlag
Berlin Heidelberg New York Tokyo

Professor Norman M. Bleehen
Department of Clinical Oncology and Radiotherapeutics
Addenbrooke's Hospital, Hills Road Cambridge, CB2 2QQ,
United Kingdom

ISBN-13: 978-3-642-69697-8 e-ISBN-13: 978-3-642-69695-4
DOI: 10.1007/978-3-642-69695-4

Library of Congress Cataloging in Publication Data.
Main entry under title:
Ovarian cancer. Collected papers of the Sixth Symposium on Clinical Oncology of the Royal College of Radiologists held Feb. 1984. Includes bibliographies and index.
1. Ovaries-Cancer-Congresses. I. Bleehen, Norman M., 1930- . II. Symposium on Clinical Oncology (6th : 1984 : London, England) III. Royal College of Radiologists (Great Britain) [DNLM: 1. Ovarian Neoplasms-congresses. WP 322 0962 1984]
RC280.08087 1984 616.99'465 85-2755

Softcover reprint of the hardcover 1st edition 1985

Typesetting, printing and binding: Appl, Wemding
2125/3140-5 4 3 2 1 0

Preface

The subject of the Sixth Symposium on Clinical Oncology of the Royal College of Radiologists held in February 1984 was ovarian cancer. This publication presents the collected papers delivered at that meeting, but excludes much useful discussion which also took place.

The annual clinical oncology symposia have been designed to review topics of current interest in cancer therapy from a multidisciplinary point if view. It was gratifying to the organisers and all who took part that the aims were so well met by both the contributors and discussants. We believe that this can only be to the advantage of future research and our present and future patients.

Ovarian cancer is a common gynaecological cancer which freqently presents late. Its clinical management is bedevilled by the variable referral routes through which patients present for treatment. Thus, many are first seen by general abdominal surgeons who may not be expert in their treatment, rather than gynaecologists or gynaecological oncologists. There are many interesting features about it which have been discussed by the various speakers. Early spread within the abdomen is common, spread outside the abdomen less common. There is a variety of histopathological types, each with distinct aetiological, prognostic and therapeutic assocations. In contrast to most cancers, surgical debulking of tumour is considered valuable even when there is no possibility of removing all tumour by the knife.

Radiotherapy has an important role in the management of both early and late disease whilst chemotherapy is rapidly finding a useful place. The questions of how best either modality should be given, whether alone or in combination, have been reviewed. Considerable excitement has been generated by the possibility of predictive testing of tumours for chemotherapy responsiveness, but a note of sensible caution was sounded at the meeting.

As with all tumours, diagnostic imaging methods are of importance. Ovarian cancer is a happy hunting ground for the exciting new imaging techniques such as computerised axial tomography and nuclear magnetic resonance that are currently becoming available. Tumour markers are available which may not only be used as an immunohistopathological guide to tumour type, or serum marker for estimation of residual or recurrent tumour mass, but now can be seen to be of value in immunoscintigraphic localisation by external radionuclide scanning. Many such exciting developments were discussed. It is hoped that this volume will therefore be of assistance and guidance to those interested in the problem of cancer of the ovary.

I wish to express my gratitude to all the speakers and discussants from the audience who enabled the symposium to proeed with vigour and interest. Finally I wish to acknowledge and thank my secretaries, Miss Lesley Sargeant and Miss Frances Rankine, for their help; Mr Michael Jackson of Springer-Verlag for his tact in understanding the problems of an editor; and Mr. A.J. Cowles and his staff at the Royal College of Radiologists for providing their excellent administrative support.

Royal College of Radiologists, London Norman M. Bleehen

Table of Contents

List of Authors

M. C. Anderson
Department of Histopathology and Colposcopy, The Samaritan Hospital for Women, London, United Kingdom

K. D. Bagshawe
Cancer Research Campaign Laboratories, Department of Medical Oncology, Charing Cross Hospital, London W6 8RF, United Kingdom

R. H. J. Begent
Department of Medical Oncology, Charing Cross Hospital, London W6 8RF, United Kingdom

V. Beral
Epidemiological Monitoring Unit, London School of Hygiene and Tropical Medicine, London WC1E 7HT, United Kingdom

M. Booth
Epidemiological Monitoring Unit, London School of Hygiene and Tropical Medicine, London WC1E 7HT, United Kingdom

K. E. Britton
Department of Nuclear Medicine, St. Bartholomew's Hospital, London EC1, United Kingdom

R. S. Bush
The Ontario Cancer Institute, The Princess Margaret Hospital, Toronto M4X 1K9, Canada

M. Granowska
Department of Nuclear Medicine, St. Bartholomew's Hospital, London EC1, United Kingdom

D. Guthrie
Regional Radiotherapy Centre, Newcastle General Hospital, Newcastle upon Tyne, United Kingdom

L. Holden
Department of Medical Oncology, Charing Cross Hospital, London W6 8RF, United Kingdom

R. J. Johnson
Department of Diagnostic Radiology, University of Manchester, and Christie Hospital and Holt Radium Institute, Manchester M20 9BX, United Kingdom

E. S. Newlands
Department of Medical Oncology, Charing Cross Hospital, London W6 8RF, United Kingdom

G. J. S. Rustin
Department of Medical Oncology, Charing Cross Hospital, London W6 8RF, United Kingdom

J. S. Scott
Department of Obstetrics and Gynaecology, Leeds University, Clarendon Wing, Leeds 2, United Kingdom

J. H. Shepherd
Department of Gynaecology, St. Bartholomew's Hospital, London EC1, United Kingdom

C. J. Williams
CRC Medical Oncology Unit, Southampton General Hospital, Southampton, United Kingdom

E. Wiltshaw
The Gynaecology Cancer Unit, Royal Marsden Hospital, London, United Kingdom

Pathology

M. C. Anderson

Department of Histopathology and Colposcopy, The Samaritan Hospital for Women, London, United Kingdom

Classification

No other organ in the human body gives rise to as many tumours as does the ovary. Because there are so many different tumours, it is essential to empoly a sensible method of classification. In these circumstances the classification is not merely a way for pathologists to make things look more complicated than they really are; it also serves the important purpose of bringing the tumours together into similar groups, outlining differences and similarities in origin, structure and, above all, behaviour.

The classification of ovarian tumours which is in use today was initiated by the International Federation of Gynecology and Obstetrics (FIGO) and further developed by the World Health Organisation (WHO) in the mid 1960s (Serov et al. 1973). It is ostensibly a classification based on histogenesis but it is, in practice, a morphological classification, with the histogenetic background being deduced from the morphological appearances. The main structures of the normal ovary from which it is believed tumours develop are: the serosa, which gives rise to the epithelial tumours; the mesenchyme, which gives rise to the sex-cord stromal tumours; and the germ cells, which give rise to the germ cell tumours. At its simplest level, therefore, the classification of ovarian tumours consists of these three groups - the epithelial tumours, the sex-cord stromal (or gonadal stromal) tumours and the germ cell tumours - each of which has many subdivisions. There are, unfortunately, some tumours which do not fit into any of these groups, mainly because their origins are not so obvious from their appearances, and these are therefore listed separately. The full classification of primary ovarian neoplasms is as shown in Table 1.

More than 90% of ovarian cancers fall into the epithelial group (Fox and Langley 1976) and these will be examined more closely, first from the point of view of tumour development. As a woman ages, the surface of the ovary becomes more corrugated, perhaps

Table 1. Primary ovarian tumours

Epithelial
Sex-cord mesenchymal
Germ cell
Lipid (lipoid) cell
Gonadoblastoma
Soft tissue tumours not specific to the ovary
Unclassified tumours
Tumour-like conditions

Ovarian Cancer, Ed. by N. M. Bleehen

as a result of ovulation, with clefts of serosa being formed, some of which may be nipped off completely, to form tiny cysts in the outer cortex. These are the very common serosal inclusion cysts and they are assumed to be the starting point for the development of most epithelial tumours of the ovary. Having stated that epithelial tumours originate from the surface epithelium, it may appear rather convoluted to take this serosa through the process of cyst formation, but these acrobatics are necessary to explain why the great majority of epithelial tumours are cystic. To appreciate the different histological types of epithelial tumour which may arise from the serosal inclusion cyst, we have to remember the embryology of the ducts of the female genital tract. The paramesonephric (Müllerian) duct is formed by direct invagination and multiplication of the coelomic lining cells. These cells will eventually form the epithelial elements of the fallopian tube, endometrium and endocervix, as well as the ectocervix and perhaps part of the upper vagina. At this very early stage of development, it is therefore apparent that these Müllerian duct cells have the ability to differentiate into all of these epithelial types. It can be argued that, if the coelomic lining cells which eventually give rise to the Müllerian duct system have these developmental competences, then adjacent coelomic lining cells on the surface of the developing ovary, and indeed the mature ovary, may be able to express the same developmental competences and differentiate along the same lines if suitably stimulated. If the epithelial lining of a serosal inclusion cyst becomes neoplastic and, as a consequence of the processes described above, differentiates along one or other cell line, then the type of epithelial tumour that results is shown in Table 2.

Although the epithelial types seen in the clear cell carcinoma and the Brenner tumour are not of Müllerian appearance, these tumours are included in the epithelial category and are usually considered to be of Müllerian origin, in that they derive from the ovarian serosa, which has been referred to as forming part of the 'secondary Müllerian system' (Lauchlan 1972). The complete list of epithelial tumours is shown in Table 3.

Of the other main groups of primary ovarian tumours, those of sex-cord stromal origin and germ cell origin are also subdivided and for the sake of completeness will be ex-

Table 2. Epithelial tumours

Fallopian tube	= Serous
Endocervix	= Mucinous
Endometrium	= Endometrioid
Mesonephric	= Clear cell
Transitional	= Brenner

Table 3. Epithelial tumours

Serous
Mucinous
Endometrioid
Clear cell
Brenner
Mixed
Undifferentiated
Unclassified

Table 4. Sex-cord stromal tumours

Ovarian differentiation (granulosa-stromal)
Granulosa cell tumour
Thecoma-fibroma
Testicular differentiation (androblastoma)
Sertoli-Leydig cell tumour (arrhenoblastoma)
Leydig cell tumour
Sertoli cell tumour

Table 5. Germ cell tumours

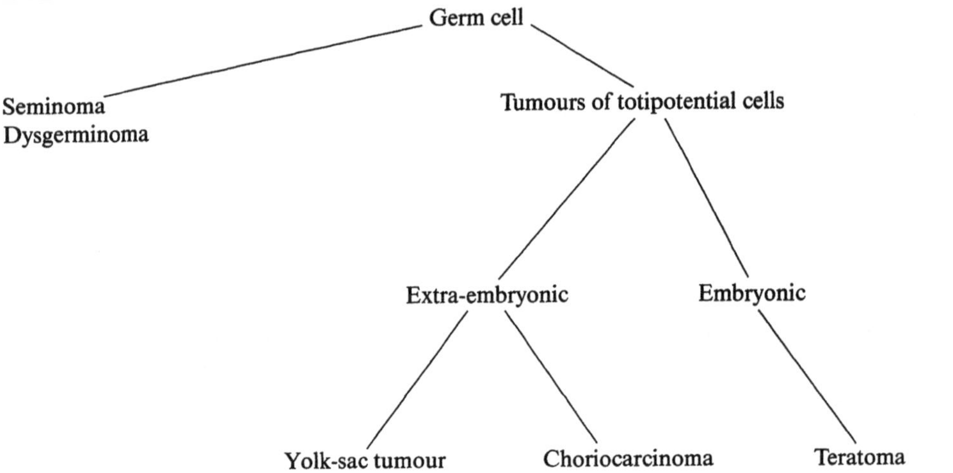

amined briefly. Table 4 shows the two major subdivisions of the sex-cord stromal tumours: those with the morphological appearance of ovarian tissue, which are usually, but not always, feminising, and those with the morphological appearance of testicular tissue, which are much rarer and are usually, but again not always, virilising. The only member of this group which is consistently malignant and therefore concerns us here is the granulosa cell tumour.

Germ cell tumours are rather more complicated and the constituent members of the group are shown in Table 5.

Surface Serous Tumours of the Ovary

As stated above, the great majority of epithelial tumours of the ovary are cystic and may develop from serosal inclusion cysts. A few tumours, however, undoubtedly do arise directly from the surface covering of the ovary and develop as exophytic, papillary growths. Tumours of this type are particularly likely to be associated with multiple pelvic and peritoneal seedlings of carcinoma. This may be expected because of the ease with which cells may break off and are then already in the peritoneal cavity without having to rupture the

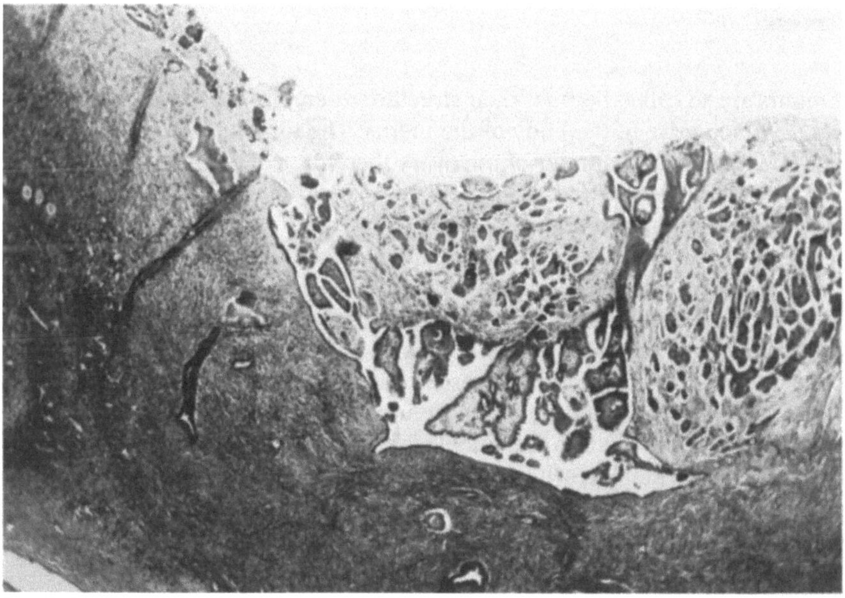

Fig. 1. Surface papillary carcinoma of the ovary (primary papillary peritoneal neoplasia). One of the numerous bilateral surface deposits of serous tumour. The omentum was also extensively involved but there was no identifiable ovarian primary tumour. H and E, × 76

capsule of the tumour. The ovarian involvement is very often bilateral. In many cases it is possible to identify one or other ovary as the site of the primary tumour, but occasionally this is not possible and the ovaries seem to be involved only by small surface deposits, indistinguishable from secondary implants (Fig. 1). These women often have quite widely disseminated intrapelvic and intraperitoneal tumour deposits, with extensive omental involvement. Although these tumours are morphologically identical to serous carcinomas it is questionable whether they should be considered as true ovarian primary tumours, and the term primary papillary peritoneal neoplasia has been coined to describe them (Foyle et al. 1981). It is argued that they probably represent a multifocal in situ neoplastic change taking place in the peritoneum generally but mainly in the pelvis, perhaps including the ovaries as part of the wider serosal change. The mechanism of histogenesis is probably the same as has been described for epithelial tumours generally. It is interesting to note that tumours of this type have been reported in women who have had prophylactic bilateral oophorectomies because of a strong familial tendency for ovarian cancer (Tobacman et al. 1982). These surface papillary tumours may be of any grade, from borderline to grade 3, but are usually stage III or IV when diagnosed. The survival of patients is shorter than that of patients with ovarian serous papillary carcinoma of the same grade without predominant surface involvement (Gooneratne et al. 1982). The recognition of this rather uncommon phenomenon explains some very puzzling histological and clinical findings in patients with serous tumours.

Endometrioid Tumours

Endometrioid tumours are so called because their structure resembles that of the primary endometrial tumours which arise in the body of the uterus. The tumour types that come under the heading of endometrioid tumour of the ovary therefore consist not only of the fairly common carcinoma but also the mesenchymal and mixed tumours. Table 6 shows a complete list of endometrioid tumours of the ovary.

Although the adenocarcinoma is the commonest member of the group, the epithelial tumours may show any of the less common epithelial patterns seen in the endometrium. Exactly what morphological features are required to enable an adenocarcinoma to be put into the endometrioid category have not been fully defined; it is not quite enough to state that any carcinoma looking like an endometrial carcinoma is an endometrioid carcinoma when found in the ovary, because an endometrial carcinoma itself may have several patterns. The basic feature of an endometrioid carcinoma is the glandular pattern, resembling the characteristic endometrial tumour, with elongated, oval or tubular glands lined by multilayered epithelium (Fig. 2). The cells do not usually contain abundant mucin but nevertheless the distinction from a mucinous carcinoma or a secondary large bowel carcinoma may not be as easy as it might seem. Many endometrioid carcinomas have papillary areas, rather more so than the endometrium, which may make their distinction from papillary serous carcinoma difficult. While on the subject of papillary carcinoma it should be stressed that papillary carcinoma of the ovary is not a precise diagnosis as papillary areas are nearly always found in serous and clear cell carcinomas, are often found in endometrioid carcinomas, and may be present in mucinous carcinomas. If the degree of differentiation allows it, which it should if the papillary pattern is well developed, the histopathologist should attempt to assign the tumour into one of these four epithelial types.

As in the endometrium, endometrioid carcinomas of the ovary may show areas of squamous metaplasia, the resultant tumour sometimes going by the name of endometrioid adenoacanthoma. The presence of malignant squamous elements in an adenosquamous carcinoma imparts a more aggressive nature to the tumour. Fu et al. (1979) reported a 5-year survival rate of only 21% in patients with adenosquamous carcinoma, compared with 90% in those with endometrioid adenoacanthoma.

The relationship of endometrioid carcinoma of the ovary to endometrial carcinoma in the body of the uterus is interesting. Up to 30% of women with endometrioid carcinomas

Table 6. Endometrioid tumours

Benign
Adenofibroma
Cystadenoma
Borderline
Malignant
Carcinoma
Adenocarcinoma
Adenoacanthoma
Adenosquamous
Endometrial stromal sarcoma
Mixed Müllerian tumours

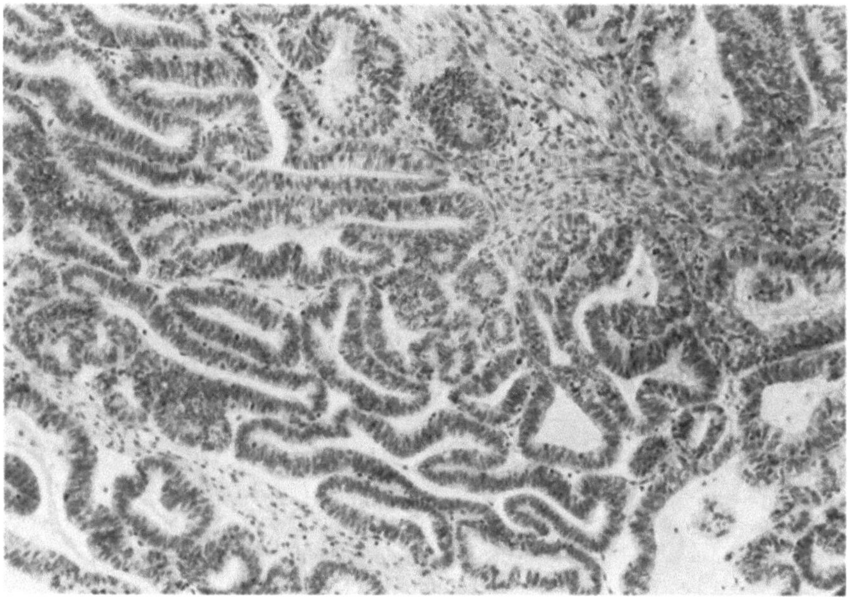

Fig. 2. Endometrioid carcinoma. The glandular pattern is similar to that seen in the commonest type of endometrial carcinoma. H and E, × 176

of the ovary are found also to have endometrial carcinomas in the uterus (Fox and Langley 1976). In a few of these cases it may be that one tumour is primary and the other is secondary, but in the majority it is believed that they represent two synchronous primary tumours. Often the ovarian tumour is large, whereas the uterine tumour is small and may be confined to the endometrium, perhaps surrounded by an area of atypical hyperplasia. Furthermore, some 10%–20% of women with endometrioid carcinomas of the ovary can be shown to have coexistent endometriosis (Czernobilsky et al. 1970). The true figure may in fact be higher, but the expansion of the tumour destroys the pre-existing endometriosis. This synchronous development of endometrioid carcinoma of the ovary and endometrial carcinoma of the uterine body may thus be regarded as a field change. The carcinogenic stimulus or stimuli is thought to have a similar effect on the endometrium in the uterus and on the ectopic endometrium in endometriosis or even upon ovarian tissue which is capable of endometrial differentiation. Finally, it should be remembered that endometrioid tumours have been found at other sites of endometriosis, away from the body of the uterus and the ovaries.

This association between an endometrioid carcinoma in the ovary and an endometrial carcinoma of the uterine body is of great importance as it means that the status of the endometrium must be assessed in all women with ovarian tumours. Although most women who are found to have malignant ovarian tumours at laparotomy will have a hysterectomy as part of the initial treatment, this is not always the case, particularly if the woman is young and the cyst is not overtly malignant at operation. In the latter circumstances, if the tumour turns out to be an endometrioid carcinoma, it is vital that the endometrium is investigated at a further operation, either by curettage or hysterectomy. An additional, perhaps rather theoretical, significance of making a correct diagnosis of endometrioid carcinoma is the possibility of progestogen sensitivity. Some endometrial carcinomas have been shown to have oestrogen and progesterone receptors, although only a minority show

Table 7. Mixed Müllerian tumours

Müllerian adenofibroma
Epithelium benign; stroma benign
Müllerian adenosarcoma
Epithelium benign; stroma malignant
Malignant mixed Müllerian tumour
Epithelium malignant; stroma malignant
Homologous
Heterologous

Table 8. Differences between ovarian malignant mixed Müllerian tumour (MMMT) and immature teratoma

MMMT	Teratoma
Older age of patient	Younger age of patient
Malignant epithelial and mesenchymal elements	Malignant epithelial elements rare
Neuroectodermal elements not seen	Neuroectodermal elements common

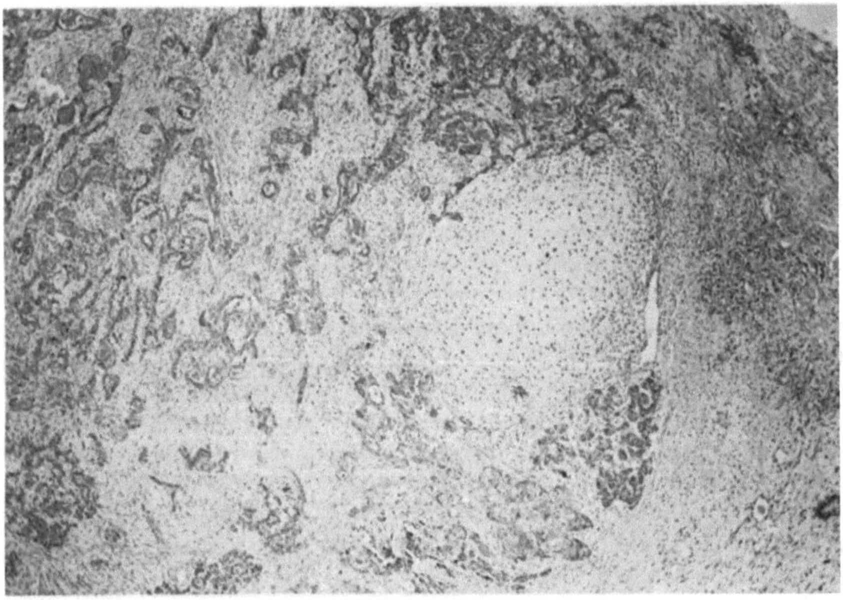

Fig. 3. Malignant mixed Müllerian tumour. Carcinomatous glands with sarcomatous stroma; a focus of chondrosarcoma is seen to the right of the centre. H and E, × 58

any clinical response to progestogen therapy. It would be expected that the morphologically identical endometrioid carcinoma of the ovary might also have progesterone receptors and so also respond to added progestogen therapy. To date, there is very little reliable information available about progesterone receptors in ovarian cancers generally, and nothing about endometrioid tumours in particular. Nevertheless, it might seem reasonable to suggest that progestogens could be added with benefit to the total treatment regimes for women with endometrioid carcinomas.

Let us now look briefly at some of the rarer variants of the endometrioid tumour - the mixed Müllerian tumours of the ovary (Table 7). These again mimic the tumours of the same name in the uterine body and are found in three degrees of malignancy. The very rare Müllerian adenofibroma is a mixture of benign mesenchymal elements and benign epithelium; the Müllerian adenosarcoma has malignant mesenchyme and benign epithelium; and the least rare malignant mixed Müllerian tumour is composed of malignant mesenchyme and malignant epithelium. The last two categories may have sarcomatous elements of homologous type, i.e. of a tissue type that would normally be found in the uterus, or they may be of heterologous type, containing tissue that would not normally be found in the uterus, such as bone, cartilage and striated muscle. Malignant mixed Müllerian tumours of heterologous type used to be called mixed mesodermal tumours; the appearance of one example is show in Fig. 3. The glandular elements are of moderately differentiated carcinoma and the mesenchymal elements contain areas of endometrial stromal sarcoma, cartilage and striated muscle. These are highly malignant tumours. The most difficult and important histological problem is to distinguish them from immature teratomas, as the malignant mixed Müllerian tumour also contains several tissue types. Sometimes this distinction can be very difficult, but the diagnosis is aided by the features listed in Table 8. The ages of women with these two tumours is different, germ cell tumours generally affecting females in the first three or four decades of life whereas malignant mixed Müllerian tumours more usually occur in women over 50. While the malignant mixed Müllerian tumour is composed of tissue which is sarcomatous and carcinomatous, the teratoma is composed of immature, embryonic, not-yet-differentiated elements. The distinction between these two types of tissue may sound straigthforward enough in theory, but in practical terms it can be very difficult to tell embryonic from sarcomatous mesenchyme. More useful in practice, perhaps, is the fact that the hallmark of the immature teratoma is presence of immature neuroepithelial elements. These are often very distinctive, but are never seen in malignant mixed Müllerian tumours.

Borderline Tumours

A few words about borderline tumours of the ovary would be appropriate, despite the fact that many would not consider them to be genuine cancers. The term borderline itself is not an altogether satisfactory one; although it is acceptable among pathologists, many gynaecologists interpret it as meaning that the pathologist is sitting on the fence and is not able to say whether the tumour is benign or malignant. The WHO classification of ovarian tumours (Serov et al. 1973) defines a borderline tumour of the ovary as one 'that has some, but not all, of the features of malignancy: those present include, in varying combinations, stratification of epithelial cells, apparent detachment of cellular clusters from their sites of origin and mitotic figures and nuclear abnormalities intermediate between those of clearly benign and unquestionably malignant tumours of a similar cell type: on the other hand, obvious invasion of the stroma is lacking'. This last feature is of the utmost importance in defining a tumour as borderline. The exclusion of invasion in the presence of epithelial atypia demands extensive and thorough sampling of the tumour, some of which, particularly those of the mucinous variety, can be very large.

Borderline tumours comprise between 8% and 15% of serous tumours of the ovary and about 20% of mucinous tumours (Ovarian Tumour Panel 1983). Examples of serous

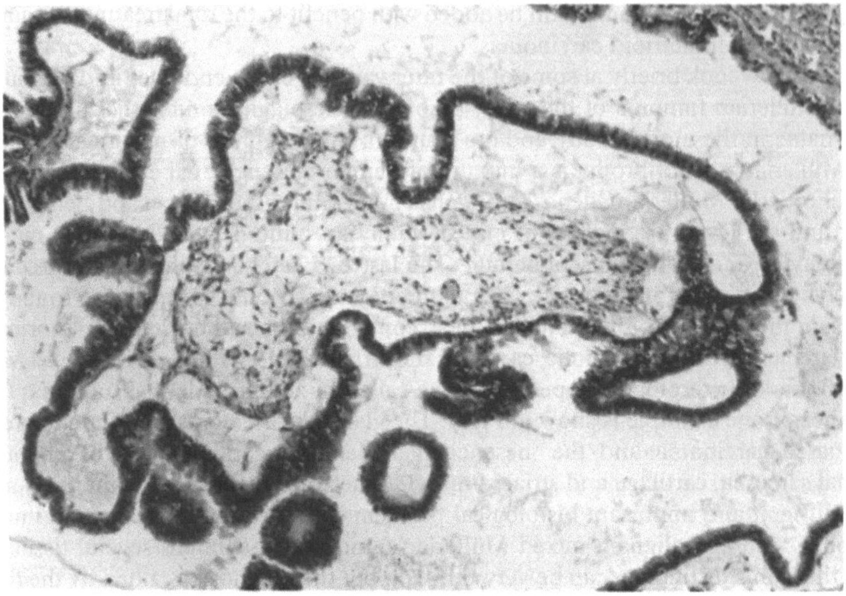

Fig. 4. Borderline serous tumour. The epithelium covering the papillae is thickened with multilayering, tufting and nuclear atypia. H and E, × 160

and mucinous borderline tumours are shown in Fig. 4 and 5. The situation is complicated by the fact that some of the tumours have extra-ovarian spread, with peritoneal deposits throughout the abdominal cavity. The deposits are usually superficial and may show the same borderline, non-invasive features as the ovarian primary tumour. In some examples, however, the extra-ovarian tumour may be of a worse histological grade than that found in the ovary. Borderline tumours of serous and mucinous types have been fairly fully described and extensively studies. However, borderline tumours of endometrioid and clear cell (mesonephroid) type and borderline Brenner tumours are sufficiently rare to remain rather obscure at present.

The reason for defining this intermediate group of ovarian epithelial tumours is that it does appear to represent a genuine subdivision which has a prognosis between that of the benign tumours and the frank carcinomas. Patients with serous borderline tumours have been reported to have a 5-year survival rate of 90%-95% (Tang et al. 1980) and a 10-year survival rate of 75%-90% (Nikrui 1981). Survival rates after 15 years have now been reported and these are in the 65%-75% range (Nikrui 1981). It is interesting to note that the mucinous borderline tumours have, on the whole, a rather poorer prognosis than the corresponding serous tumours. This is in contrast to the relative prognoses of the respective carcinomas, perhaps suggesting that some mucinous carcinomas may be erroneously diagnosed as borderline.

These results indicate that, even if energetic treatment is not justified immediately for borderline tumours, long-term follow-up must be maintained. Some would advocate that the therapy should be no less radical than for an unquestionably malignant tumour of the same stage (Ovarian Tumour Panel 1983). Nevertheless, borderline tumours present a number of dilemmas. Tumours of identical histological appearance and stage can behave in strikingly different ways, some apparently advancing very indolently, if at all, over many years, while others lead to the death of the patient in a short time. It may be that

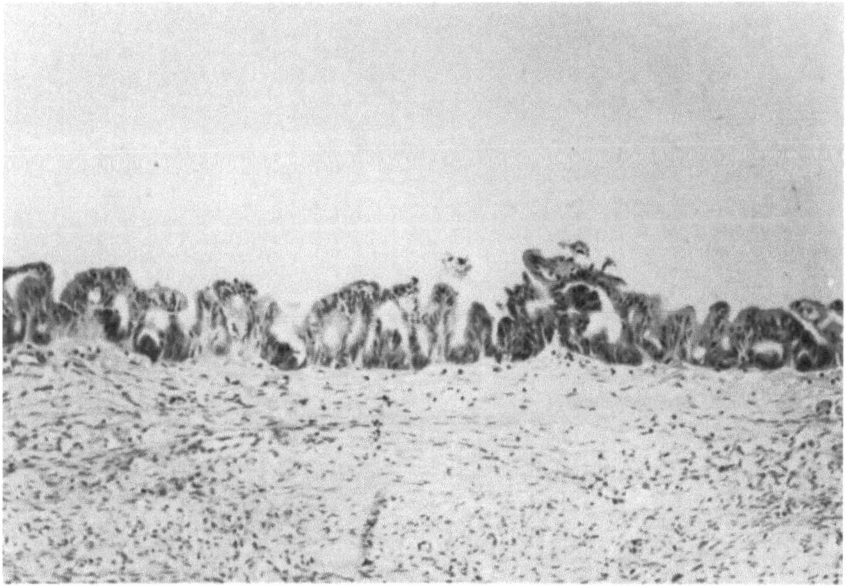

Fig. 5. Borderline mucinous tumour. The features of the epithelium are rather more pronounced than in Fig. 4. H and E, × 154

some borderline tumours will remain as such for years, while others will rapidly develop into frankly malignant tumours. In the latter case the borderline tumours may merely be an early phase in the development of malignancy. There is a need for more extensive studies of borderline tumours in an attempt to define prognostic features more precisely.

Grading

The assessment of ovarian cancer covers three broad categories. The first, which is a clinical exercise, is staging. The other two are both histological, and involve determining the histological type of the tumour and its grade. Although there are differences in the behaviour of malignant tumours according to the histological type, as for example between a yolk-sac tumour and mucinous carcinoma, within the group of common epithelial tumours, the grade of the tumour is probably a more useful indicator of aggressiveness than the histological type (Sorbe et al. 1982).

To most histopathologists, grading is simply a matter of putting the tumour into one of three categories: well differentiated, moderately differentiated and poorly differentiated. The problem is, however, a little more complicated than this, because the architectural pattern and the nuclear appearances should be assessed separately. Architectural grading is judged for adenocarcinomas in general according to how closely the tumour resembles the normal tissue from which it has arisen. This is straightforward enough for endometrium, colon or stomach, but makes less sense in the ovary where the tumours have not arisen from pre-existing glandular structures. A modification of Broders' grading system is used, in which the proportion of cells contributing to gland formation is estimated. The grade 1 tumours have most cells (over 75%) contributing to glands, whereas the grade 3 tumours have a few cells (less than 25%) forming glands, with expanses of solid sheets of tu-

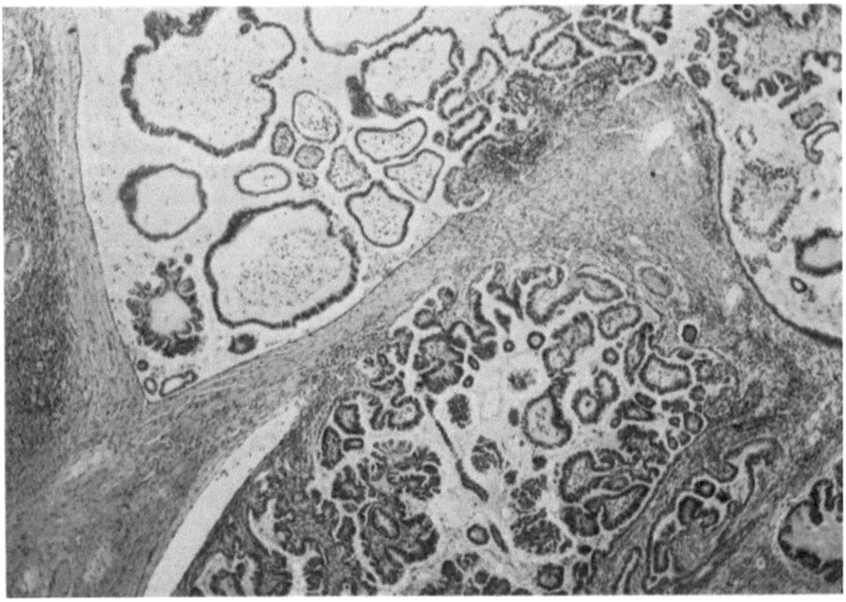

Fig. 6. Papillary serous carcinoma, architectural grade 1. Almost all the neoplastic epithelial cells are contributing to the covering epithelium. H and E, × 62

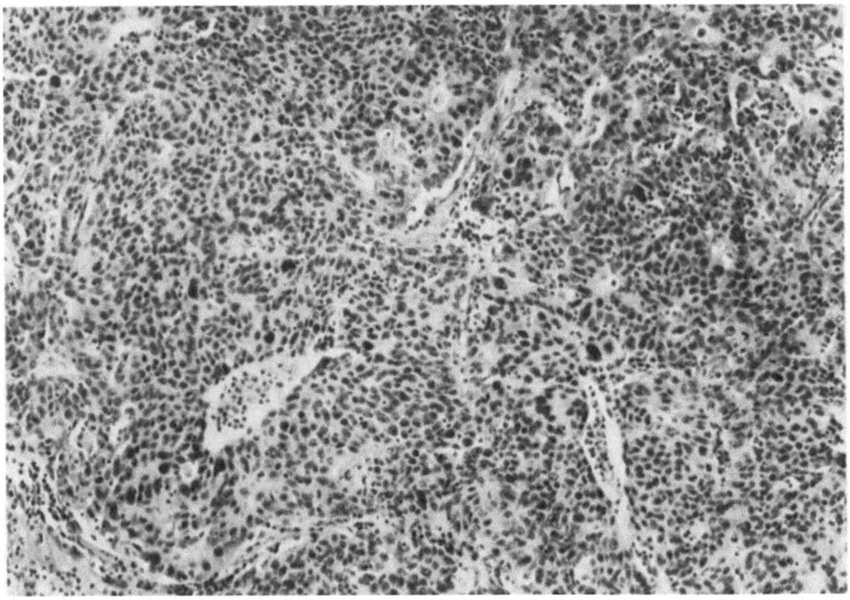

Fig. 7. Papillary serous carcinoma, architectural grade 3. The tumour cells form solid masses, with very few glandular spaces. The diagnosis of the histological type has to be made from other, better differentiated areas. H and E, × 180

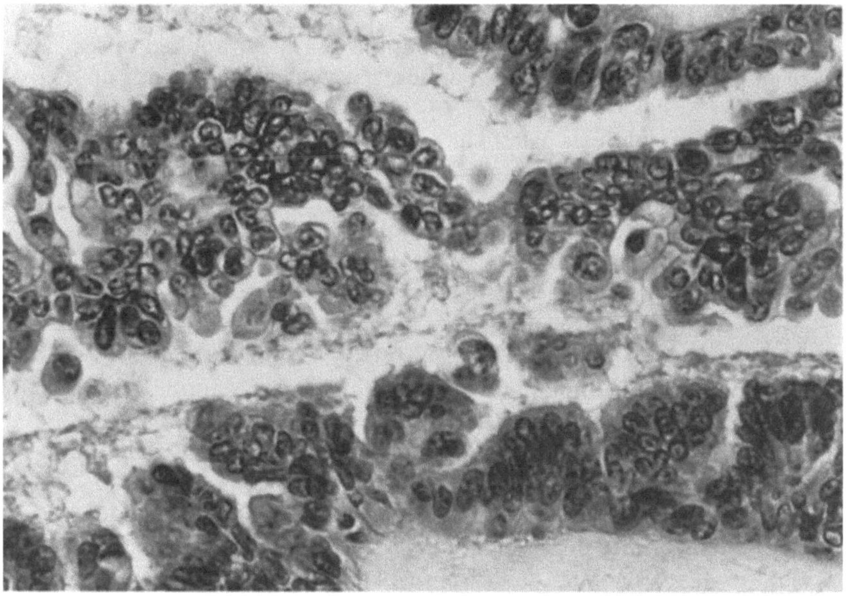

Fig. 8. Papillary serous carcinoma, nuclear grade 1. Although enlarged, the nuclei are fairly regular and are not hyperchromatic. No mitotic figures are seen in this field. H and E, × 590

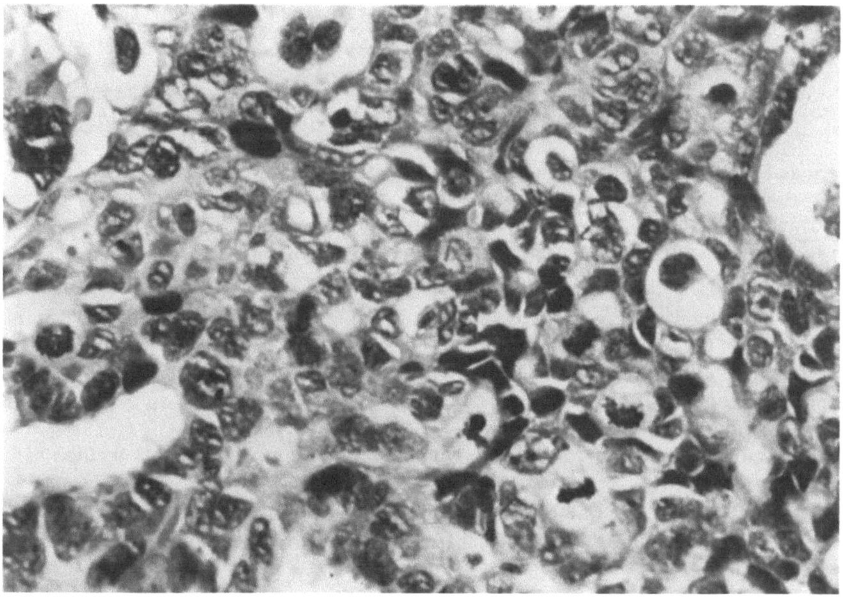

Fig. 9. Papillary serous carcinoma, nuclear grade 3. There is marked variation in nuclear size and shape with hyperchromasia. Mitotic figures are numerous. The histological type cannot be determined from this field. H and E, × 590

mours cells (Fig. 6 and 7). These criteria are easy enough to apply to endometrioid and mucinous tumours, where gland formation is expected, but are less easily applied to serous tumours, which are mainly papillary, or clear cell tumours, which have solid and papillary components.

Nuclear grading disregards the glandular pattern and concentrates on the nucleus and its relationship to its own cell and other nuclei. Such features as the nuclear-cytoplasmic ratio, nuclear pleomorphism, variation in size and mitotic activity are taken into account (Fig. 8 and 9). Although in the majority of instances the architectural grade and nuclear grade of a tumour correspond, this is not always so and, if the two grades differ, it is the nuclear grade which is the more significant as regards tumour behaviour.

These comments apply to the grading of the common epithelial tumours and not necessarily to other tumours. For example there is no evidence that the architectural pattern or nuclear appearances of granulosa cell tumour have any bearing on its prognosis, which is related more to stage than any other assessable feature. Different criteria are used for other tumours; for example, immature teratomas are usually graded according to the proportion of immature neuroepithelial tissue present.

The existence of these three assessable features - stage, histological type and grade - causes problems for anyone embarking on a comparative study of ovarian cancer, its treatment and behaviour, because very large numbers of patients must be included to achieve valid numbers in any one category. For the epithelial tumours there are four histological types, each with four stages and a minimum of three grades in each stage, which gives a possible total of 48 individual subgroups. However, it seems that for grade 3 tumours the histological type is largely immaterial as the patients all fare uniformly badly.

References

Czernobilsky B, Silverman BB, Mikuta JJ (1970) Endometrioid carcinoma of the ovary: a clinicopathological study of 75 cases. Cancer 26: 1141-1152

Fox H, Langley FA (1976) Tumours of the ovary. Heinemann, London

Foyle A, Al-Jobi M, McCaughey WTE (1981) Papillary peritoneal tumors in women. Am J Surg Path 5: 241-249

Fu YS, Stock RJ, Reagan JW, Storaalsi JP, Wentz WB (1979) Significance of squamous components in endometrioid carcinoma of the ovary. Cancer 44: 614-621

Gooneratne S, Sassone M, Blaustein A, Talerman A (1982) Serous surface papillary carcinoma of the ovary: a clinicopathologic study of 16 cases. Int J Gynecol Pathol 1: 258-269

Lauchlan SC (1972) The secondary Müllerian system. Obstet Gynecol Surv 27: 133-146

Nikrui N (1981) Survey of clinical behaviour of patients with borderline epithelial tumors of the ovary. Gynecol Oncol 12: 107-119

Ovarian Tumour Panel of the Royal College of Obstetricians and Gynaecologists (1983) Ovarian epithelial tumours of borderline malignancy: pathological features and current status. Br J Obstet Gynaecol 90: 743-750

Serov SF, Scully RE, Sobin LH (1973) Histological typing of ovarian tumours. International histological classification of tumours no 9. World Health Organisation, Geneva

Sorbe B, Frankendal B, Veress B (1982) Importance of histological grading in the progress of epithelial ovarian carcinoma. Obstet Gynecol 59: 576-582

Tang M, Lian L, Liu T (1980) The characteristics of ovarian serous tumours of borderline malignancy. Chin Med J 92: 450-464

Tobacman J, Greene MH, Tucker M, Costa J, Kase R, Fraumani JF (1982) Intra-abdominal carcinomatosis after prophylactic oophorectomy in ovarian-cancer-prone families. Lancet II: 795-797

Occurrence and Aetiology

V. Beral and M. Booth*

Epidemiological Monitoring Unit, London School of Hygiene and Tropical Medicine, London WC1E 7HT, United Kingdom

Distribution of Ovarian Cancer

Each year nearly 4500 new cases of ovarian cancer are diagnosed in England and Wales and over 3500 women die from the condition (Office of Population Censuses and Surveys 1983 a, b). There are now more deaths from ovarian cancer each year than from cancers of the uterine cervix and corpus combined. One reason for the relatively large number of ovarian cancer deaths is the high case fatality rate. In England and Wales only 25% of women with the malignancy survive as long as 5 years after diagnosis. With such a depressingly poor prognosis, one slightly encouraging feature is that younger women do survive longer than older patients. For example, 41% of those who are 35-44 years old at diagnosis survive for 5 years, compared with 17% of those aged 65-74 (Office of Population Censuses and Surveys 1981).

The prominence of ovarian cancer as a cause of death in women today is of concern as there has been a substantial increase in its incidence over the past 70 years (Office of Population Censuses and Surveys 1981). It can be seen from Fig. 1 that the age-adjusted annual mortality rate has doubled in about 50 years from around 7 per 100000 women in 1926-30 to 14 per 100000 in 1976-80. Part of the apparent increase may be due to improvements in diagnosis over the years; but some is almost certainly real. In contrast to ovarian cancer, mortality from cancer of the uterine cervix has been falling, as has (until, perhaps, recently) mortality from endometrial cancer. Breast cancer rates have, somewhat surprisingly, remained relatively stable throughout the 70-year period. Not only is the incidence of ovarian cancer increasing in England and Wales, but similar trends are evident in other countries for which information is available (Beral et al. 1978). Furthermore it is more common in developed than developing countries, the highest incidence rates being reported from Sweden and Norway, the lowest from Japan and other Asian countries (International Agency for Research on Cancer 1976). Within any one country, rates are highest in the professional classes and lowest in the unskilled (Beral et al. 1978).

Incidence and mortality rates increase rapidly with age, until the sixth decade, after which they begin to plateau (Fig. 2). Similar age trends have been described for all the main histological types of epithelial ovarian tumours and also for sex-cord and mesenchymal tumours (Weiss et al. 1977). Only germ cell tumours differ in their age pattern, with dysgerminomas occurring predominantly around the age of 20 years, and malignant teratomas showing a bimodal age distribution. One of these peaks occurs before the age of 30 years, and is followed by a progressive increase in incidence at older ages (Berg and

* We thank Helen Edwards for typing the manuscript

Ovarian Cancer, Ed. by N. M. Bleehen

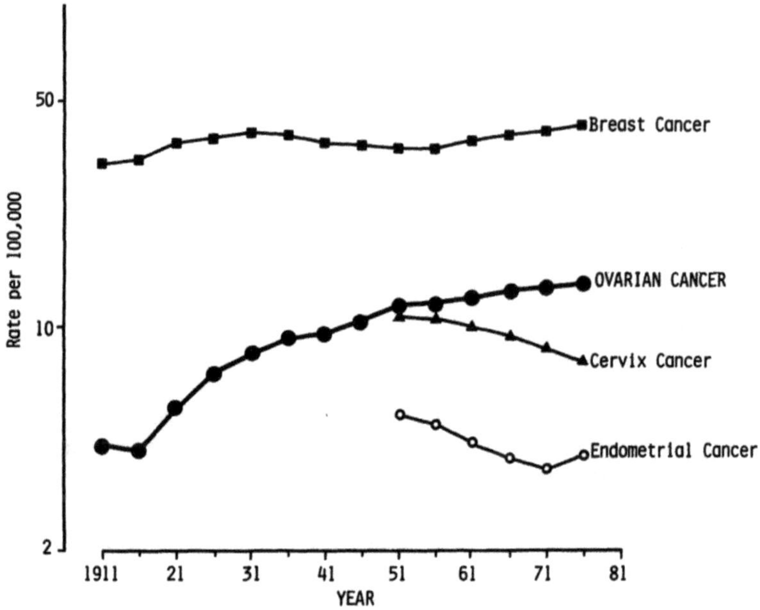

Fig. 1. Trends in age-adjusted mortality rates per 100000 women for ovarian cancer, breast cancer, and cancers of the uterine cervix and endometrium. England and Wales. 1911-78

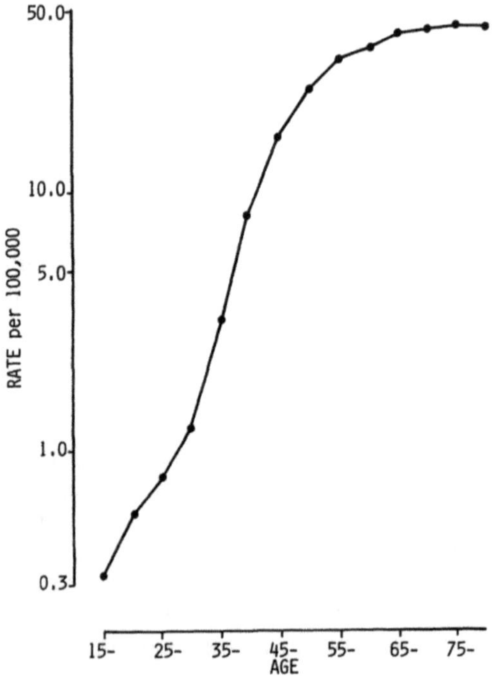

Fig. 2. Age-specific mortality rates per 100000 women for ovarian cancer. England and Wales, 1975-79

Baylor 1973). The slight deflection of the age-specific mortality rates at 20–24 years seen in Fig. 2 probably represents the relatively high proportion of germ cell tumours at that age. In older age groups epithelial tumours dominate.

Little is known about trends or international variation in the occurrence of the various histological types of ovarian tumours. Such studies are hampered by differences in diagnostic criteria used over time or from place to place. Bearing in mind such problems, Berg and Baylor (1973) suggested that there may be a close geographical similarity in the distribution of adenocarcinomas of the ovary, granulosa cell tumours and malignant teratomas. Only dysgerminomas show a different geographical distribution.

Familial, Genetic and Ethnic Factors

Familial factors are important in determining susceptibility to ovarian cancer. Women whose mother or sister had the disease have almost a 20-fold increase in the risk of acquiring the malignancy themselves (Hildreth et al. 1981; Franceschi et al. 1982). Inheritance is mainly reported to be through the maternal line, but paternal inheritance has also been described (Matheson et al. 1981). It is, of course, not possible to know whether this strong familial clustering represents genetic susceptibility or shared exposure to an environmental factor. Women with ovarian cancer are also more likely to have a family history of cancer of the uterine corpus, but not of breast cancer (Hildreth et al. 1981). Despite this strong familial tendency, 95% of women with ovarian cancer do not have a family history of the disease (Hildreth et al. 1981; Franceschi et al. 1982).

Although a family history of breast cancer is not associated with an increased risk of ovarian cancer, women who had breast cancer in their premenopausal years are at a considerably increased risk of developing ovarian cancer (Prior and Waterhouse 1981). This may, however, reflect environmental influences rather than common susceptibility to the two conditions. Women with rare conditions such as the Peutz-Jegher syndrome or chromosomal abnormalities have also been reported to be at an increased risk of ovarian cancer. Turner's syndrom and other anomalies of the sex chromosomes have been associated mainly with the development of germ cell tumours (Pfeiffer et al. 1983). Ovarian cancer has also been linked with blood group A (Osborne and De George 1963).

Ethnic differences in ovarian cancer incidence are not great. Japanese, Chinese, Hispanio and black women living in the United States have similar incidence of non-epithelial tumours to white women, but have slightly lower rates of all the major epithelial tumour types (Weiss and Peterson 1978). Thus the large geographic differences in ovarian cancer incidence are probably explained by environmental, rather than ethnic factors (Beral et al. 1978).

Hormones, Reproduction and Ovulation

In the last 5 years a number of studies have reported on the association of ovarian cancer with reproduction, menstrual history and the use of exogenous hormones (e.g. Casagrande et al. 1979; Hildreth et al. 1981; Risch et al. 1983). In collaboration with Dr. P. G. Smith, we are carrying out a study based in London and Oxford investigating the relationship of these factors to ovarian cancer. In general, a number of consistent findings

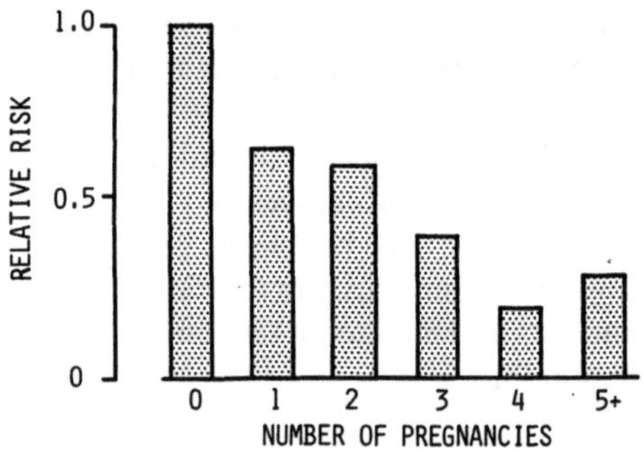

Fig. 3. Relative risk of ovarian cancer by number of pregnancies

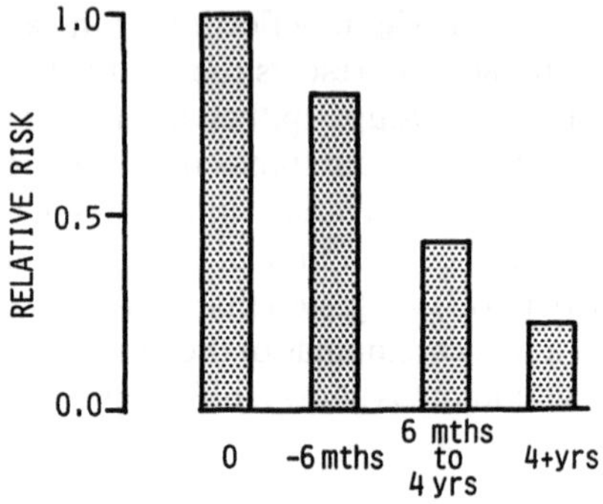

Fig. 4. Relative risk of ovarian cancer by duration of oral contraceptive use

have emerged. The first is that nulliparous women are at an increased risk of developing the disease compared with parous women. It is still unclear, however, whether these women are nulliparous by choice or whether infertility plays a part in the aetiology of the disease. Another consistent finding is that the risk of acquiring the disease declines progressively with the number of children a woman has had. This is illustrated by our data in Fig. 3. It can be seen that women with one pregnancy have a risk of ovarian cancer approximately half that of women who have had no pregnancies, and women with four or more pregnancies have approximately a quarter the risk. Not only does a full-term pregnancy confer protection from disease, but so does an incomplete one (Casagrande et al. 1979). An early age at menarche and a late age at menopause are also associated with an increased risk of the disease. Risch et al. (1983) found that breastfeeding is an additional protective factor.

Oral contraceptives also appear to protect women from ovarian cancer. This finding was first reported by Newhouse et al. in 1977, and has since been replicated many times. Our results, shown in Fig. 4, are consistent with those already reported, and show that the protection is greater the longer the pill is taken. In contrast to oral contraceptives, the use of oestrogens for menopausal symptoms has been reported to be associated with increased risk of ovarian cancer, especially endometrioid and clear cell tumours (Hoover et al. 1977; Cramer et al. 1981; Weiss et al. 1982). These findings have not been confirmed by all investigators.

The general observation that the risk of ovarian cancer is reduced by any method which suppresses ovulation, or lessens the number of ovulations a woman experiences during her life, supports Fathalla's hypothesis (1971) that incessant ovulation is an important factor in the aetiology of ovarian cancer. There are, however, some difficulties with the interpretation of this hypothesis. For example, the effects of ovulation suppression by just one pregnancy or a few months' use of oral contraceptives (see Fig. 3 and 4) are perhaps larger than might be expected (La Vacchia et al. 1983; Rich et al. 1983). The mechanism by which ovulation might induce carcinogenesis is also unclear; for example, is repeated trauma of the surface of the ovary during ovulation important, or do cyclical hormonal changes promote tumour growth?

Environmental Factors

Asbestos

In 1960, Keal suggested that women with asbestosis had increased rates of ovarian cancer. Since then studies of women exposed to asbestos at work have reported an increase in the rates of ovarian cancer (Acheson et al. 1982; Wignall and Fox 1982). There remains, however, a question about the validity of the diagnosis in certain cases. Some abdominal mesotheliomas may have been wrongly classified as primary ovarian cancer. Despite serious attempts to confirm the diagnoses, it is clear that it is often impossible to know precisely from where a tumour first arose. Furthermore, pathologists disagree on the criteria used to differentiate between mesothelioma and primary ovarian cancer.

Talc

Interest in talc as a possible carcinogen began when Henderson et al. (1971) observed that a high proportion of ovarian tumours had talc particles embedded in them. This observation is of interest since talc can be contaminated with asbestos, a substance already implicated as a possible ovarian carcinogen. In 1982 Cramer et al. described that women with ovarian cancer were twice as likely as controls to use talc as a dusting powder in the perineal region or on sanitary towels. Since then, Hartge et al. (1983) have reported no association between the use of talc in general and ovarian cancer, but they did note that women with ovarian cancer were more likely than controls to use talc in the genital area. This difference was not, however, statistically significant. These observations, while far from clear cut, do suggest that talc may be a factor in the aetiology of ovarian cancer.

Ionising Radiation

There is now considerable evidence that ionising radiation is carcinogenic to a number of tissues in humans. Forty years ago it was not uncommon to treat certain benign gynaecological conditions, such as metropathia haemorrhagica, with pelvic irradiation. Follow-up studies of women thus treated have shown that they were subsequently at an increased risk of developing cancers in the pelvic region (Smith 1977).

Pelvic Surgery

Two studies (Annegers et al. 1979, Hildreth et al. 1981) reported that women who have had a hysterectomy may have a reduced incidence of ovarian cancer. The meaning of these findings is, however, not immediately obvious. The relevant factor may be either a suppression of ovulation caused by the hysterectomy, or the removal of ovaries at the time of operation if suspicious, premalignant changes are present. Finally the observations may be biased, as it may not always have been possible to establish whether a woman's ovaries had or had not been conserved at the time of hysterectomy.

Prophylactic oophorectomy is sometimes recommended for women in families with a strong propensity to ovarian cancer. Tobacman et al. (1982) reported, however, that 3 out of 28 women so treated developed intra-abdominal tumours. Although the primary site was uncertain, these tumours were histologically indistinguishable from ovarian cancer. They suggested that cancer-prone families may have potentially malignant tissue not only in the ovary, but in the coelomic epithelium.

Infections

In 1966, West noted that women with ovarian cancer were less likely to report having had mumps than were matched controls. Newhouse et al. (1977) repeated his observation, also noting that women with ovarian cancer were less likely to report having had other childhood infections.

Serological studies have yielded conflicting results, but Menczer et al. (1979) reported that women with ovarian cancer were more likely to have developed subclinical mumps and to have lower titres of mumps-complement-fixing antibodies. Cramer and his colleagues (1983) found an inverse relationship between age at menarche and menopause in women with a history of mumps but not in women without a history of mumps, suggesting that the mumps virus may determine reproductive span. Contrary to other investigators, they suggested that mumps might increase ovarian cancer risk.

Diet

Because ovarian cancer is a disease of mainly Western societies, it has been suggested that diets characteristic of the West, such as high consumption of animal fats, may be important in the aetiology of the malignancy. A systematic survey of the diet of women with ovarian cancer has recently been reported by Byers et al. (1983). They found no clear association between ovarian cancer and consumption of fats, protein, vitamin C, alcohol or tea. They did note, however, that ovarian cancer patients aged 30–49 years were less likely than controls to consume diets rich in fibre or vitamin A. They did not confirm the observation of Trichopoulos et al. (1981) that coffee consumption may increase the risk of ovarian cancer.

Conclusions

Not only is the incidence of ovarian cancer increasing, but survival remains poor. Although a number of factors which may protect against the disease have now been identified, many are not of immediate practical relevance. For example, even though it has been established that the risk of ovarian cancer decreases with increasing parity, the present custom of having small families is unlikely to be influenced by the observations. Furthermore, even if oral contraceptives are protective, caution is needed since oral contraceptives might also enhance the risk of other cancers (Pike et al. 1983). It is interesting, nevertheless, that mortality rates from ovarian cancer are falling in women under 50 years of age (Fig. 5), and this may be due to women of that age having used oral contraceptives in the past.

Even if the possibilities for the primary prevention of ovarian cancer are still unclear, secondary prevention, that is the detection and treatment of preclinical malignant disease,

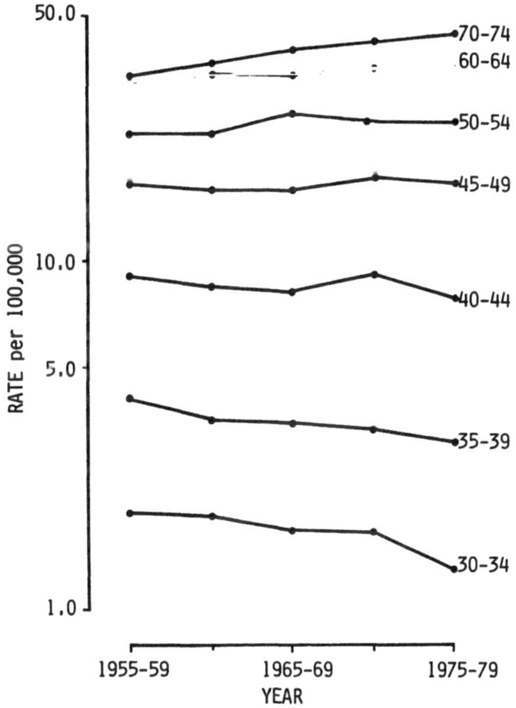

Fig. 5. Trends in selected age-specific mortality rates per 100000 women for ovarian cancer. England and Wales, 1955-79

may be feasible. Campbell et al. (1982) have reported on the possible use of ultrasound as a screening procedure. It remains to be seen whether this approach will be useful in lessening the burden of fatal ovarian cancer in the community.

Summary

Ovarian cancer is mainly a condition of industrialised societes. Its incidence is increasing, and in England and Wales more women now die from ovarian cancer than from cancers of the uterine cervix and corpus combined. A number of recent studies have highlighted the role of incessant ovulation in the aetiology of ovarian cancer: the more times a woman ovulates in her reproductive life, the greater is her risk of ovarian cancer. For example, factors suppressing or preventing ovulation - pregnancy, oral contraceptive use, or early menopause - lessen a woman's risk of developing ovarian cancer. Although the evidence is not always consistent, other factors reported possibly to reduce the risk of ovarian cancer include hysterectomy, a diet high in fibre and vitamin A, and a past history of mumps. Factors which may increase the risk include working with asbestos, dusting the genital area with talc, and exposure of the pelvic area to ionising irradiation.

References

Acheson ED, Gardner MJ, Pippard EC, Grime LP (1982) Mortality of two groups of women who manufactured gas masks from chrysotile and crocidolite asbestos: a 40-year follow up. Br J Indust Med 39: 344-348

Annegers JF, Strom H, Decker DG, Dockerty MB, O'Fallon WM (1979) Ovarian cancer. Incidence and case-control study. Cancer 43: 723-729

Beral V, Fraser P, Chilvers C (1978) Does pregnancy protect against ovarian cancer? Lancet I: 1083-1087

Berg JW, Baylor SM (1973) The epidemiologic pathology of ovarian cancer. Hum Pathol 4: 537-547

Byers T, Marshall J, Graham S, Mettlin C, Swanson M (1983) A case-control study of dietary and non-dietary factors in ovarian cancer. J Natl Cancer Inst 71: 681-686

Campbell S, Goessens L, Goswamy R, Whitehead M (1982) Real-time ultrasonography for determination of ovarian morphology and volume. A possible screening test for ovarian cancer? Lancet I: 425-426

Casagrande JT, Pike MC, Ross RK, Louie EW, Roy S, Henderson BE (1979) Incessant ovulation and ovarian cancer. Lancet II: 170-173

Cramer DW, Welch WR, Cassalls S, Scully RE (1983) Mumps, menarche, menopause and ovarian cancer. Am J Obstet Gynecol 147: 1-6

Cramer DW, Welch WR, Scully RE, Wojciechowski CA (1982) Ovarian cancer and talc. A case-control study. Cancer 50: 372-376

Cramer DW, Devesa SS, Welch WR (1981) Trends in the incidence of endometrioid and clear cell cancers of the ovary in the United States. Am J Epidemiol 114: 201-208

Fathalla MF (1971) Incessant ovulation: A factor in ovarian neoplasia? Lancet II: 163

Franceschi S, La Vecchia C, Mangioni C (1982) Familial ovarian cancer: Eight more families. Gynecol Oncol 13: 31-36

Hartge P, Hoover R, Lesher LP, McGowan L (1983) Talc and ovarian cancer. J Am Med Assoc 250: 1844

Henderson WJ, Joslin CAF, Turnbull AC, Griffiths K (1971) Talc and carcinoma of the ovary and cervix. J Obstet Gynaecol Br Cwlth 78: 266-272

Hildreth NG, Kelsey JL, LiVolsi VA, Fischer DB, Holford TR, Mostow ED, Schwartz PE, White C (1981) An epidemiology study of epithelial carcinoma of the ovary. Am J Epidemiol 114: 398-405

Hoover R, Gray LA Sr, Fraumeni JF (1977) Stilboestrol (Diethylstilboestrol) and the risk of ovarian cancer. Lancet II: 533-534

International Agency for Research on Cancer (1976) Cancer incidence in five continents, vol 3. IARC Scientific Publication No. 15. IARC, Lyon

Keal EE (1960) Asbestosis and abdominal neoplasms. Lancet II: 1211-1216

La Vecchia C, Franceschi S, Gallus G, Decarli A, Liberati A, Tognoni G (1983) Incessant ovulation and ovarian cancer: A critical approach. Int J Epidemiol 12: 161-164

Matheson JAB, Matheson H, Anderson SA (1981) Familial ovarian cancer. How rare is it? J R Coll Gen Pract 31: 743-745

Menczer J, Modan M, Ranon L, Golan A (1979) Possible role of mumps virus in the aetiology of ovarian cancer. Cancer 43: 1375-1379

Newhouse ML, Pearson RM, Fullerton JM, Boesen EAM, Shannon HS (1977) A case control study of carcinoma of the ovary. Br J Prev Soc Med 31: 148-153

Office of Population Censuses and Surveys (1981) Cancer statistics: incidence, survival and mortality in England and Wales. Studies on Medical and Population Subjects 34: 76-77

Office of Population Censuses and Surveys (1983a) Cancer statistics: registrations. Series MB1 No. 11. HMSO, London

Office of Population Censuses and Surveys (1983b) Mortality statistics: cause. Series DH2 No. 9. HMSO, London

Osborne RH, De George FV (1963) The ABO blood groups in neoplastic disease of the ovary. Am J Hum Genet 15: 380-388

Pfeiffer RA, Tietze U, Krone HA, Schaaff A, Dhom G, Peter H (1983) Invasive dysgerminoma in a girl with 45 × solidus, 46 × Mar Mosaicism. Arch Gynecol 233: 141-147
Pike MC, Henderson BE, Krailo MD, Duke A, Roy S (1983) Breast cancer in young women and use of oral contraceptives: possible modifying effect of formulation and age at use. Lancet II: 926-930
Prior P, Waterhouse JAH (1981) Multiple primary cancers of the breast and ovary. Br J Cancer 44: 628-636
Risch HA, Weiss NS, Lyon JL, Daling JR, Liff JM (1983) Events of reproductive life and the incidence of epithelial ovarian cancer. Am J Epidemiol 117: 128-139
Smith PG (1977) Leukaemia and other cancers following radiation treatment of pelvic disease. Cancer 39: 1901-1905
Tobacman JK, Tucker MA, Kase R, Greene MH, Costa J, Fraumeni JF Jr (1982) Intra-abdominal carcinomatosis after prophylactic oophorectomy in ovarian-cancer-prone families. Lancet II: 795-797
Trichopoulos D, Papapostolou M, Polychronopoulou A (1981) Coffee and ovarian cancer. Int J Cancer 28: 691-693
Weiss NS, Homonchuk T, Young JL (1977) Incidence of the histologic types of ovarian cancer: the US Third National Cancer Survey, 1969-1971. Gynecol Oncol 5: 161-167
Weiss NS, Peterson AS (1978) Racial variation in the incidence of ovarian cancer in the United States. Am J Epidemiol 107: 91-95
Weiss NS, Lyon JL, Krishnamurthy S, Dietert SE, Liff JM, Daling JR (1982) Non-contraceptive oestrogen use and the occurrence of ovarian cancer. J Natl. Cancer Inst 68: 95-98
West RO (1966) Epidemiologic study of malignancies of the ovaries. Cancer 19: 1001-1007
Wignall BK, Fox AJ (1982) Mortality of female gas mask assemblers. Br J Ind Med 39: 34-38

Surgery

J. S. Scott

Department of Obstetrics and Gynaecology, Leeds University, Clarendon Wing, Leeds 2, United Kingdom

Introduction

The role of surgery in the diagnosis and management of ovarian cancer has undergone great changes in the past decade and continues to change. Not all the new approaches have been universally accepted or applied, so there exists a state of transition compounded by some confusion.

There are a number of inherent reasons for the problems. The surgical approaches recommended are in many respects contrary to accepted principles of cancer surgery. Many cases present with abdominal symptoms and/or signs which do not specifically point to a gynaecological lesion. So, unlike the situation with any other gynaecological cancer, the primary surgery is often performed by a general surgeon, frequently a junior one, who may have little knowledge of recent developments in relation to ovarian cancer. It is also possible that the initial operation is done on the presumption of there being a benign gynaecological mass by a gynaecologist who is not familiar with current policies for cancer. It is to be hoped that the more widespread availability of efficient imaging techniques, particularly ultrasound, will reduce the frequency of operations performed without the diagnosis having been made or strongly suspected. There will continue to be, however, patients operated on by surgeons on an acute basis when admission has been for abdominal pain, in whom the cause of the pain is shown ultimately at laparotomy to be due to torsion, rupture or haemorrhage in a cancerous ovarian tumour. Whatever the reason for it happening, an operation done by a surgeon inexpert in the field is likely to be unsatisfactory with regard to staging, and the excision inadequate.

These remarks apply to primary surgery and such problems tend not to arise with secondary surgery. Such secondary surgery is often referred to by the unsatisfactory term 'second-look laparotomy', which covers a variety of surgical approaches having in common only the fact that they are planned procedures. This is an aspect concerning which there is much difference of opinion, with some surgeons seeking any excuse to perform such procedures, others any excuse to avoid them. Most of these comments apply to the common category of primary surface epithelial tumours of a definitely invasive nature occurring in women of mature years. There are special considerations with regard to some rare tumours, particularly the germ cell cancers, which usually present in relatively young women.

Ovarian Cancer, Ed. by N. M. Bleehen

Primary Surgery

The aims of primary surgery are (1) confirmation of suspected diagnosis; (2) staging of the extent of disease; (3) curative operations; and (4) incomplete or debulking operations to improve the prospects of success for chemotherapy or radiotherapy.

Confirmation of Diagnosis

The pre-operative suspicion of ovarian cancer may be based upon the clinical history and examination, the imaging findings and sometimes cytology of ascitic fluid. Rarely the hint comes from the reporting of malignant cells thought to be of ovarian origin in a cervical smear. At operation appearances are all too often typical of a frankly cancerous lesion with spread to other tissues. The finding of malignant cells on cytology at operation will augment the clinical observation as, of course, does frozen-section histology.

Staging of Disease

Unlike most cancers the staging of ovarian cancer is primarily an operative procedure. The realisation that staging errors were the probable reason for the very poor results obtained with early ovarian cancers which had been apparently adequately treated surgically has led to a much more meticulous approach to staging laparotomy. It was reported (Bagley et al. 1973; Rosenoff et al. 1975) that in cases previously surgically staged as Stage I or II, subdiaphragmatic metastases could frequently be demonstrated by laparoscopy. In addition it came to be appreciated that there was also the possibility that metastases in the omentum, para-aortic and pelvic lymph nodes could be missed and that malignant cells in peritoneal washings constituted another indication of tumour spread which had frequently been overlooked. A combination of these factors accounts for the very poor results with apparent stage I and II cases (Piver 1983 a).

The practical importance of these points for the surgeon are that (1) he must open any abdomen possibly containing ovarian cancer through a vertical incision; (2) if an apparently localised malignant tumour is discovered the incision should be extended above the umbilicus to allow full abdominal evaluation; (3) the diaphragm should be inspected and any suspicious nodules sampled (laparoscopic biopsy forceps may be used for this purpose); (4) saline should be injected into the paracolic gutters, the pelvic and subdiaphragmatic areas to be re-collected for cytological examination; (5) omentectomy should be performed to allow detailed search for microscopic metastases; (6) any enlarged para-aortic or pelvic nodes should be biopsied; (7) both large and small bowel should be carefully inspected as well as other peritoneal surfaces and biopsies taken as appropriate; and (8) he should ensure that adequate operating time is available to allow careful performance of all these procedures.

If there is thought to be any question of surgery involving bowel resection pre-operative preparation of the bowel is appropriate. Prediction in these matters is so difficult that many surgeons adopt it as a routine measure whenever ovarian cancer is the suspected diagnosis.

Curative Operations

The conventional surgery aimed at cure for stage I and II cases used to be removal of the ovaries together with the fallopian tubes and uterus. The appreciation of the frequency of macroscopically undetectable omental metastases has led to that basic surgery being extended to include removal of the omentum as routine. This should, of course, be part of the staging procedure but it is also of therapeutic value.

In a group of stage II patients with fixed pelvic tumours and without major disease above the umbilicus, the operation of radical oophorectomy has been advocated by Hudson (1968, 1981); Howkins and Hudson (1983). The aim is to mobilise the pelvic peritoneum, approaching it from behind the rectum, and having incised it and freed it round the pelvic brim to use it as a false capsule in which to remove the whole tumour. The pelvis is left devoid of peritoneum. This approach relies heavily upon the low invasiveness of many ovarian tumours on the serosal surface.

Incomplete or Debulking Operations

The greatest change with regard to surgery in ovarian cancer in recent years has been in the treatment of those tumours which are not removable by a block surgical excision, particularly those of stage III. It had come to be appreciated that ovarian cancer which had spread beyond the limits of effective surgical excision could, following chemotherapy, be compatible with quite significant 5-year survival times if there was no gross residual disease (Day and Smith 1975). It was reported that only 2% of 323 patients were surviving at 5 years if the largest remaning lesion was over 1 cm in diameter, whereas around 30% survived 5 years if the largest remaining lesion was 1 cm or less (Day and Smith 1975). Such observations led to a much more radical approach even when the tumour was not excisable *en masse*. The aim of surgery became to remove, if at all possible, the uterus, both fallopian tubes and ovaries together with the omentum, and to reduce all tumour masses in the abdomen to a size of around 1 cm in diameter or less. This can be a difficult and tedious surgical task which may not appeal to the surgeon who sees himself in the role of curer and finds it an approach contrary to basic surgical principles. However, for the surgeon who has insight into his contemporary role as a member of the team managing a cancer problem it is one which can be appreciated as worthwhile.

Obviously the findings in advanced cases can be of such a varied nature that no precise rules can be laid down and an *ad hoc* approach has to be adopted. Exploration of the upper abdomen to exclude gastric or colonic primary growth should be performed at an early stage, for if it is found that such is the basis of the neoplasia and the ovarian masses are secondary then the surgical strategy becomes entirely different. It is important for the surgeon to appreciate that even when ovarian cancer has spread widely within the abdomen there may have been very little invasion. Frequently tumour masses covering extensive serosal surfaces, including bowel, can be removed by gentle blunt dissection without damaging the underlying structure or producing serious haemorrhage. Where the liver parenchyma is involved, however, there is little to be gained from proceeding to such cytoreductive surgery, as the prognosis is unlikely to be improved.

Secondary Surgery

For secondary (or second-look) surgery the abdomen is re-opened either very soon after the initial operation (early) or after a course of relatively prolonged cytotoxic therapy (late).

Early

Early operation is done, for example, when primary surgery has been by modern standards inadequate for accurate staging or the extent of surgical excision has been less than optimal. In practice it can be very difficult to decide whether any real or theoretical deficiencies in the original surgery are sufficient to justify submitting the unfortunate patient to a second laparotomy within a few days or weeks. Better staging, while very important in improving the quality of studies on ovarian cancer, will not necessarily improve the prognosis for the individual; it can make it appear worse if the classification comes to be changed from stage I to stage III. A more radical therapeutic regime may be used because of more advanced staging, but careful thought as to what may or may not be done depending on possible new findings may make it clear that it is not necessarily in the interests of the individual to perform immediate repeat laparotomy. A compromise arrangement may sometimes give the patient the best, or the least bad, of both worlds. For example, if using 6 or 12 months of chemotherapy followed by late second-look laparotomy is contemplated, then precise knowledge as to whether the stage is I or III at the outset need not affect the initial treatment. Subsequent management would depend on the findings at the later operation, thus avoiding an early second-look procedure.

Similar difficulties exist when the adequacy of excision is in doubt, though here one can be certain that the patient's own interest is the only factor. It still remains a matter of fine judgement whether or not to operate again after a very short interval.

Late (After Chemotherapeutic Treatment)

If a patient with ovarian cancer has had apparently successful chemotherapeutic treatment there is often still doubt as to whether or not the tumour has been completely eradicated. None of the modern imaging techniques will detect very small neoplastic deposits in the peritoneal cavity. To avoid further unnecessary, unpleasant and, in the long term, potentially dangerous cytotoxic treatment (Reimer et al. 1977; Curry et al. 1981; Webb et al. 1982), re-exploration of the abdomen is advocated. There is no firm agreement as to when re-operations should be done. Piver (1983b) concludes from his experience that second-look laparotomy should be performed after 12 monthly cycles of chemotherapy. Given a negative secondary laparotomy of adequate extent, prolonged survival seems to occur in about 70% cases (Schwartz and Smith 1980; Curry et al. 1981; Roberts et al. 1982).

The procedure at laparotomy demands full evaluation of the diaphragm, para-aortic and pelvic nodes, omentum, intestine and other abdominal contents, plus peritoneal washings, as at the initial staging. The procedure is, in effect, a re-staging. Multiple peritoneal biopsies are recommended, with particular attention to areas where tumour was recorded as being present initially.

In addition to confirming the absence of active intraperitoneal disease the second laparotomy may allow resection of any tumour masses of significant size; such masses may have been present and unresectable at the time of initial operation. The value of secondary debulking procedures has, however, been questioned (Raju et al. 1982; Jacobs et al. 1983). Any acute complications may indicate a secondary laparotomy at any time after the initial treatment, but confusion arises if these operations are referred to as second-looks.

The use of laparoscopy with biopsies and/or peritoneal washing cytology has been advocated to reduce the incidence of repeated laparotomy. If the laparoscopy demonstrates cancer then laparotomy may be pointless, but if laparoscopy is negative, and the aim is to prove as far as possible that no cancer remains after therapy, then it is necessary to proceed to laparotomy.

One reason for the lack of enthusiasm for second-look procedures on the part of some surgeons is that there is a rate of false negative explorations as high as 30% (Mangioni et al. 1979). Random peritoneal biopsy is obviously a haphazard and unscientific approach while cytology on peritoneal washings is also a problem as after therapy the cellular appearances can be highly misleading. Furthermore, second-look tends to lead to third-look etc. (Copeland et al. 1983) and rationality demands some limit.

Surgery for Borderline Malignancy in Young Women

The essential criterion of borderline malignancy of ovarian tumours is the presence of malignant epithelium associated with no stromal invasion. Borderline ovarian malignancy is an exception to the general rules of surgical approaches to cancer, at least as regards the management of relatively young women who do, or may in the future, desire to have children. Borderline tumours occur most frequently in women between 20 and 40 years of age (Piver 1983b). The initial optimal procedure is oophorectomy or salpingo-oophorectomy on the affected side. If frozen-section findings suggest a tumour of borderline malignancy then longitudinal wedge biopsy of the other ovary is appropriate to exclude neoplasm there. If that is negative and full staging exploration reveals no sign of tumour elsewhere then preservation of reproductive function is a reasonable option. The initial histology report may inevitably require revision in the light of more extensive microscopy performed at leisure which demands a histology block for every 1–2 cm of tumour.

Management of borderline ovarian cancer is still evolving, but on current evidence no adjuvant therapy appears indicated in stage I cases, though careful follow-up is clearly necessary (Katzenstein et al. 1978; Julian and Woodruff 1972; Piver 1983b). Expansion of the present relatively meagre information on the natural history of borderline ovarian cancer may well lead to modification of current surgical approaches.

Ovarian Tumours in Pregnancy

Symptomless ovarian tumours are not infrequently discovered in pregnancy as a result of vaginal examinations or ultrasound scans done at the outset. There are a number of reasons for operating on such cases in the course of pregnancy but the major one is the risk of the tumour being malignant and the deterioration in prognosis likely to result from delaying operation until the post-partum phase. Standard practice has been to delay operation until the second trimester. By this time the corpus luteum ceases to be responsible for the hormonal support of the pregnancy so sacrifice of the corpus luteum, if it happens to be on the tumour-bearing ovary, is unlikely to disturb the pregnancy. However, efficient ultrasound scanning can now indicate with a high degree of confidence if an ovarian mass is purely a cystic one. Absence of a demonstrable solid component makes it very unlikely that it will prove malignant. Accordingly, current practice in this matter is in a state of transition, with a proportion of women with ovarian tumours in pregnancy having their operations postponed until after delivery. Deciding factors are the quality of the ultrasound and the size of the tumour.

Place of Ovarian Cystectomy

Most British gynaecological surgeons practising today have been exposed in their training to the Victor Bonney philosophy of conservative surgery in relation to ovarian cysts and uterine fibroids. This continues to have much to commend it but there is some confused thinking about the procedures. Occasional tragedies occur if enucleation is performed on an ovarian tumour which turns out to be malignant and the consequence is metastatic spread. If there is any suggestion of a significant solid component to a unilateral ovarian mass then cystectomy is *not* an appropriate operation. This approach is greatly assisted today by efficient ultrasound scanning. The correct procedure, if there is a solid component to the mass, is oophorectomy or salpingo-oophorectomy. This will be most unlikely to result in spread from disturbance of the tumour if it is cancerous. Also there should be little or no risk of reduction of fertility as all subsequent gonadotrophin pulses will tend to induce ovulation in the remaining ovary. If a further solid tumour does develop in the remaining ovary then fertility will almost certainly have to be sacrificed, but such a sterilising form of surgery would be indicated even if a portion of the first ovary had been retained initially.

Germ Cell Tumours in Young Women

Germ cell cancers of the ovary are relatively unimportant numerically, accounting for only around 10% of ovarian cancers. However, without the best of modern treatment they may carry a very high mortality. They also particularly afflict young females before or soon after reaching child-bearing age, so their significance is far greater than their numbers. They represent a great challenge in deciding therapy, with the need to balance survival prospects against preservation of fertility. For long, radical surgical approaches were followed and augmented by radiation and chemotherapy. However, in a number of series it was reported that dysgerminoma, the commonest of the germ cell tumours, had been managed by unilateral salpingo-oophorectomy, despite the fact that dysgerminoma has a high incidence of bilateral occurrence. Lucraft (1979) reported on 12 stage Ia cases; 4 given post-operative radiation showed no recurrence while of 8 not given radiation, 4 recurred but responded to radiation subsequently. Put another way, managed by this method all the women were tumour free but for one-third their fertility had been preserved.

Asadourian and Taylor (1969) also point to a high response rate of recurrences to radiotherapy; in their series there was a recurrence in 10 of 46 cases after unilateral salpingo-oophorectomy. Boyes et al. (1979) reported a series of patients with dysgerminoma seen between 1938 to 1976 in which from 1960 there was a policy change from unilateral salpingo-oophorectomy to pelvic clearance preceding radiation. This new approach was followed by complete success in terms of lack of recurrence. However, this policy change was contrary to that which others have been making. Developments in chemotherapy and tumour marker assay employed in combination carry the prospect of cure with preservation of reproductive function and are leading to more conservative approaches to unilateral germ cell tumours (Scott 1983).

The appropriate surgical approach to germ cell ovarian neoplasms can be summarised as:

1. High awareness of the possibility of germ cell cancer in young females with clinical solid ovarian neoplasms.
2). Appropriate arrangements for frozen-section and cytological studies at operation. The histology should be done on removal of the ovarian mass intact, not by biopsy.
3. A provisional decision before operation as to whether a conservative line will be followed if a unilateral germ cell cancer confined to the ovary is found.
4. If there are such findings at laparotomy, then unilateral (salpingo-)oophorectomy with full staging procedures should be performed. While the frozen-section examination is undertaken, the contralateral gonad should be inspected closely and a wedge biopsy performed.

Evidence is accumulating that individual treatment according to the precise type of histology can be of great importance in the management of germ cell tumours. This is contrary to the position with the surface epithelial tumours, in which the histological type has little bearing, at least on the initial management. It is not too strong to say that improved chemotherapeutic approaches combined with monitoring of response by tumour marker measurement are revolutionising management in the field of germ cell tumours. Good responses occur even in cases in which there is already metastatic spread (Newlands et al. 1982). Wiltshaw et al. (1982) recorded complete remission in 7 or 8 cases of endodermal sinus (yolk-sac) tumour treated with conservation of the uterus and an ovary. Pregnancies have been recorded after treatment of various germ cell tumours (Forney 1978; Duncan and Young 1980). In other cases regular menstruation has been recorded following successful treatment, indicating that ovulation is probably occurring normally. The overall picture in regard to child-bearing after chemotherapeutic management appears to be good. Though conception rates are reduced there is no evidence of a substantial increase in pregnancy wastage or fetal abnormality (Barber 1981).

Sixty-seven of a series of 72 (93%) patients with stage Ia pure dysgerminoma treated by unilateral salpingo-oophorectomy were alive and disease-free at 5 years (Gordon et al. 1981). Weinblatt and Ortega (1982) advocate giving chemotherapy initially for extensive dysgerminoma in childhood in the hope that extensive surgery which will destroy fertility can be avoided.

The aim with germ cell tumours has been summarised as to 'achieve maximal cure rate with minimal sterilisation rate' (Scott 1983). Whatever views one may have about centralisation of cancer care in general, there is a very strong case indeed for the management of these rare germ cell tumours in young women being centralised in a few units where special expertise exists concerning all aspects of care.

Surgery in the Prevention of Ovarian Cancer

Oophorectomy at Hysterectomy for Benign Indications

Oophorectomy at hysterectomy is a potential but in some respects controversial role for surgery in the prevention of ovarian cancer. Many women in Western societies have hysterectomy performed for indications other than malignancy. Obviously such operations bring an opportunity to remove the ovaries. 'No ovaries, no ovarian cancer' is the simplistic view, but the widespread removal of benign ovaries from a large proportion of women is something which requires profound consideration from many points of view. At present there is little agreement on surgical practice.

When hysterectomy is being performed after the natural menopause then it is usual to remove both ovaries on the grounds that they have ceased endocrine function yet still may become cancerous. In a younger woman an ovary which looks unhealthy will usually be excised but beyond that policies at hysterectomy vary widely. Surprisingly, considering the importance of the issue on a numerical and personal basis, there are very few data available upon which to base a rational policy decision.

An unexpected finding in one excellent but small-scale study on the place of oophorectomy when hysterectomy is being performed for benign indications (Annegers et al. 1979) was that women who had undergone hysterectomy but with preservation of both ovaries apparently had a reduced incidence of ovarian cancer. Other studies have supported the idea that surgical menopause when done by hysterectomy without oophorectomy is beneficial (Wynder et al. 1969; Joly et al. 1974; McGowan et al. 1979; Cramer et al. 1983). The possibilities are (1) that these women represent a special low-risk section of the population; (2) that removal of the uterus carries a benefit by some mechanism hitherto quite unsuspected, or (3) that the mere fact that the ovaries were conserved at the time of hysterectomy indicated that they were particularly healthy in appearance and unlikely to become cancerous. As mentioned above, it is common to remove an ovary when its appearance is in any way suggestive of actual or potential neoplasia, so it seems quite probable that this last effect operates (Cramer et al. 1983).

It is possible that if one ovary is removed randomly at hysterectomy this reduces the cancer risk (Annegers et al. 1979; Cramer et al. 1983) without incurring any unwanted effects, as the remaining ovary will continue to produce steroid hormones. Theoretically this depends on the method of carcinogenesis operating. If it is incessant ovulation as proposed by Fathalla (1971) then removal of one ovary would not be expected to reduce cancer incidence - possibly the reverse. If it is assumed that approximately 50% of ovulations occur in each ovary, then after unilateral oophorectomy 100% of ovulations would be in the remaining ovary and therefore likely to boost its chance of becoming cancerous. If, on the other hand, in this cancer of relatively advanced age the development is dependent upon random gene mutation in the tissue mass, reducing the mass by 50% could be expected to reduce the cancer risk by up to this amount. Until more worthwhile data are available, surgeons are likely to continue individualised policies based upon prejudices and direct personal experience. Gathering information on this important matter should be a top priority at present. It is a chastening thought that at present many a gynaecological surgeon's contribution to the ovarian cancer problem - positive or negative - may be an entirely thoughtless, fortuitous one!

Excision of Dysgenetic Gonads

There is a small but very important and widely agreed place for prophylactic surgery in relation to germ cell tumours. It has long been known that intersexual individuals of female phenotype have a significantly raised chance of malignant germ cell tumours occurring at a very early age. More recently this has been refined to indicate that the major risk, a high one of the order of 25%, is in individuals with dysgenetic gonads or asymmetric gonadal differentiation who possess a Y chromosome. This occurs often as part of an XO/XY or XX/XY mosaic or chimaeric chromosome constitution (Schellhas 1974a, b; Scott 1985). The commonest tumour is a gonadoblastoma. Most of these cases will have been diagnosed clinically as Turner's syndrome or pure gonadal dysgenesis. These unfortunate individuals have no realistic prospect of reproductive function and even ovarian steroid hormone production is not likely to occur. So the existence of this very high risk makes excision of the dysgenetic gonads not only reasonable but mandatory. The operation should be performed as soon as the combination of an XY cell line and the presence of one or more dysgenetic gonads is established in a phenotypic female. Fig. 1 illustrates the findings of a gonadal tumour on one side of the pelvis and a streak, dysgenetic gonad on the other. The tumour proved to be a dysgerminoma which was ultimately fatal nearly 15 years after the initial operation. The patient proved to have an XX/XY chromosome constitution which was of chimaeric rather than mosaic origin, the evidence being that two sperms had been involved in the conception (Bain and Scott 1965). Such a tumour could almost certainly be prevented nowadays by full investigation of the intersexual state at an early age and prompt prophylactic surgery.

There is also some increased risk of gonadal malignancy in intersexual individuals lacking an XY cell line. The order of risk in such cases is not nearly so high and almost

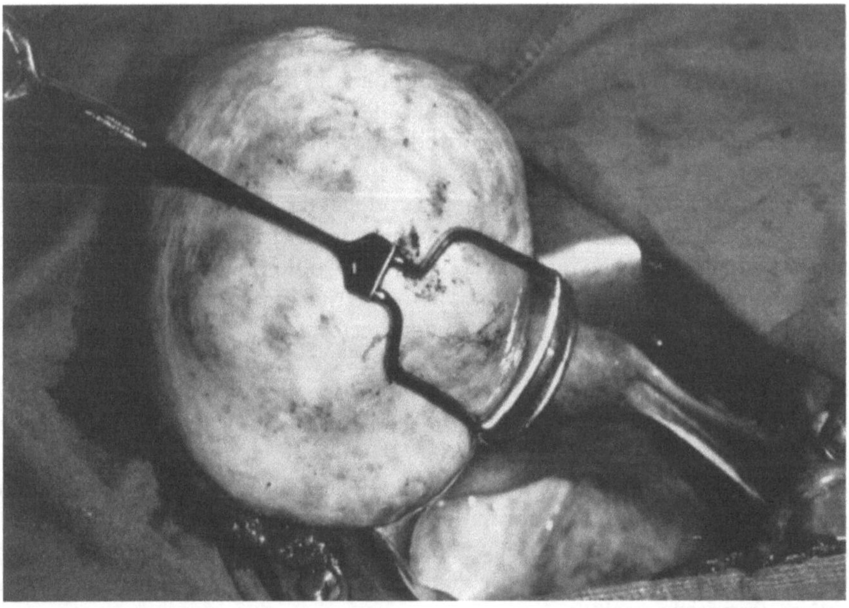

Fig. 1. Unilateral ovarian tumour. On the opposite side can be seen a typical streak gonad. The tumour proved to be a dysgerminoma and the patient was found to be an XX/XY chimaera. Death occurred from metastases almost 15 years after primary surgery

certainly not of a sufficient order to justify prophylactic surgery on all such cases. The development of techniques for detection of the HY antigen offered a prospect of identifying the individuals at high risk, but this has not yet been realised (Scott 1985).

Excision of Gonads in Androgen Insensitivity Syndrome

Phenotypic females with an XY sex chromosome complement who have some form of the androgen insensitivity or testicular feminisation syndrome are also at risk of gonadal neoplasia and prophylactic gonadal excision has a place. However, the nature, degree and age incidence of the risk are quite different from those associated with streak or dysgenetic gonads. Neoplasia, often benign, occurs in 3%-6% of these individuals before 25 years of age, rising to 33% at 50 years. Although child-bearing is not possible, the hormonal production is frequently effective in producing desirable female secondary sex characteristics. Postponement of prophylactic operation until about 25 years of age seems reasonable (Manuel et al. 1976; Scott 1985).

Patients with a Strong Familial Tendency to Ovarian Cancer

There may be rare families, such as those with the Peutz-Jeghers syndrome (which consists of microcutaneous pigmentation with intestinal polyposis: Fox and Langley 1976), in which the incidence of ovarian cancer is so high that at some age gonadal excision seems justified.

Summary

From this short review it can be seen that optimal surgery for ovarian cancer has changed in recent years, but many patients still have traditional surgery. Many operations are not done by gynaecologists because the diagnosis has not been made, but modern scanning techniques are capable of improving this. Primary surgery involves diagnosis, staging, attempted cure and debulking procedures. A long vertical incision is essential. Secondary (or second-look) surgery may be done 'early', if the initial operation has been unsatisfactory, or 'late', after chemotherapeutic treatment, to confirm remission or for other indications.

Special problems exist with borderline malignancy, and with ovarian tumours in pregnancy and in young women, particularly when germ cell cancer is suspected.

There is also a potential prophylactic role for surgery (1) in relation to hysterectomy which is being performed for non-malignant indications, when one or both ovaries may be removed, and (2) in intersexual individuals of the types known to be associated with a high risk of gonadal malignancy, when dysgenetic gonads should be excised.

References

Annegers JF, Strom H, Decker DG, Dockerty MB, O'Fallon WM (1979) Ovarian cancer. Incidence and case-control study. Cancer 43: 723-729

Asadourian LA, Taylor HB (1969) Dysgerminoma: An analysis of 105 cases. Obstet Gynecol 33: 370-379

Bagley CM Jr, Young RC, Schein PS et al. (1973) Ovarian carcinoma metastatic to the diaphragm frequently undiagnosed at laparotomy. A preliminary report. Am J Obstet Gynecol 116: 397-400

Bain AD, Scott JS (1965) Mixed gonadal dysgenesis with XX/XY mosaicism. The evidence for the occurrence of fertilisation by two spermatozoa in man. Lancet I: 1035-1039

Barber HRK (1981) The effect of cancer and its therapy upon fertility. Int J Fertil 26: 250-259

Boyes DA, Pankratz E, Galliford BW et al. (1979) Experience with dysgerminomas at the cancer control agency of British Columbia. Gynecol Oncol 6: 123-129

Copeland LJ, Wharton JT, Felix FN, Gershenson DM, Seski JC, Herson J (1983) Role of 'third-look' laparotomy in the guidance of ovarian cancer treatment. Gynecol Oncol 15: 145-153

Cramer DW, Hutchison GB, Weich WR, Scully RE, Ryan KJ (1983) Determinants of ovarian cancer risk.I. Reproductive experiences and family history. J Natl Cancer Inst 71: 711-716

Curry SL, Zembo MM, Nahas WA, Jahshan AE, Whitney CW, Mortel R (1981) Second-look laparotomy for ovarian cancer. Gynecol Oncol 11: 114-118

Day TG, Smith JP (1975) Diagnosis and staging of ovarian carcinoma. Semin Oncol 97: 217-222

Duncan ID, Young JL (1980) Endodermal sinus tumour of the ovary: Serum alpha-fetoprotein levels before and after treatment and during pregnancy. Br J Obstet Gynaecol 87: 535-538

Fathalla MF (1971) Incessant ovulation: A factor in ovarian neoplasia? Lancet II: 163

Forney JP (1978) Pregnancy following removal and chemotherapy of ovarian endodermal sinus tumour. Obstet Gynecol 52: 360-362

Fox H, Langley FA (1976) Tumours of the ovary. Heinemann, London

Gordon A, Lipton D, Woodruff JD (1981) Dysgerminoma: A review of 158 cases from the Emil Noval Ovarian Tumor Registry. Obstet Gynecol 58: 497-504

Howkins J, Hudson CN (1983) Radical oophorectomy. In: Shaw's textbook of operative gynaecology, 5th edn. Churchill Livingstone, Edinburgh London, pp 321-324

Hudson CN (1968) A radical operation for fixed ovarian tumours. J Obstet Gynaecol Br Cwlth 75: 1155-1160

Hudson CN (1981) Ovarian cancer: A gynaecological disorder? Ann R Coll Surg Engl 63: 118-125

Jacobs AJ, Kubitz RL, Scott JC, Kessinger MA (1983) Surgery following initial treatment of ovarian carcinoma: Restaging (second-look) and palliative operations. J Surg Oncol 24: 59-63

Joly DJ, Lilienfield AM, Diamond EL, Bross ID (1974) An epidemiologic study of the relationship of reproductive experience to cancer of the ovary. Am J Epidemiol 99: 190-209

Julian CG, Woodruff JD (1972) The biologic behaviour of low grade papillary serous carcinoma of the ovary. Obstet Gynecol 40: 860-867

Katzenstein ALA, Mazur MT, Morgan TE, Kao MS (1978) Proliferative serous tumours of the ovary. Am J Surg Pathol 2: 339-355

Lucraft HH (1979) A review of thirty-three cases of ovarian dysgerminoma emphasizing the role of radiotherapy. Clin Radiol 30: 585-589

McGowan L, Parent L, Lednar W, Norris HJ (1979) The woman at risk for developing ovarian cancer. Gynecol Oncol 7: 325-344

Mangioni C, Bolis G, Molteni P, Belloni C (1979) Indications, advantages and limits of laparoscopy in ovarian cancer. Gynecol Oncol 7: 47-55

Manuel M, Katayama KP, Jones HW (1976) The age of occurrence of gonadal tumors in intersex patients with a Y chromosome. Am J Obstet Gynecol 124: 293-300

Newlands ES, Begent RHJ, Rustin GJS, Bagshawe KD (1982) Potential for cure in metastatic ovarian teratomas and dysgerminomas. Br J Obstet Gynaecol 89: 555-560

Piver MS (1983 a) Staging laparotomy in stage I and II ovarian malignancies. In: Singer A, Jordan J (eds) Ovarian malignancies: The clinical care of adults and adolescents. Current reviews in obstetrics and gynaecology 4. Churchill Livingstone, Edinburgh London, pp 74-82

Piver MS (1983 b) Borderline ovarian carcinomas. In: Singer A, Jordan J (eds) Ovarian malignancies: the clinical care of adults and adolescents. Current reviews in obstetrics and gynaecology 4. Churchill Livingstone, Edinburgh London, pp 68-73

Raju KS, McKinna JA, Barker GH, Wiltshaw E, Jones JM (1982) Second-look operations in the planned management of advanced ovarian carcinoma. Am J Obstet Gynecol 144: 650-654

Reimer RR, Hoover R, Fraumeni FF et al. (1977) Acute leukemia after alkylating-agent therapy of ovarian cancer. N Engl J Med 297: 177-181
Roberts WS, Hodel K, Rich WM, DiSaia PJ (1982) Second-look laparotomy in the management of gynecologic malignancy. Gynecol Oncol 13: 345-355
Rosenoff SH, De Vita VT Jr, Hubbard S et al. (1975) Peritoneoscopy in the staging and follow-up of ovarian cancer. Semin Oncol 2: 223-228
Schellhas HF (1974a) Malignant potential of the dysgenetic gonad: I. Obstet Gynecol 44: 298-309
Schellhas HF (1974b) Malignant potential of the dysgenetic gonad: II. Obstet Gynecol 44: 455-462
Schwartz PE, Smith JP (1980) Second-look operations in ovarian cancer. Am J Obstet Gynecol 138: 1124-1130
Scott JS (1983) Rays of hope for rare ovarian cancers. Br Med J 286: 824-825
Scott JS (1985) Intersex and sex chromosome abnormalities. In: RR Macdonald (ed) Scientific basis of obstetrics and gynaecology (3rd ed). Churchill Livingstone, Edinburgh London, pp 201-254
Webb MJ, Snyder JA, Williams TJ, Decker DG (1982) Second-look laparotomy in ovarian cancer. Gynecol Oncol 14: 285-293
Weinblatt ME, Ortega JA (1982) Treatment of children with dysgerminoma of the ovary. Cancer 49: 2608-2611
Wiltshaw E, Stuart-Harris R, Barker GH, Gowing NFC, Raju S (1982) Chemotherapy of endodermal sinus tumour (yolk sac tumour) of the ovary: Preliminary communication. J R Soc Med 75: 888-892
Wynder EL, Doder H, Barber HR (1969) Epidemiology of cancer of the ovary. Cancer 23: 352-370

Tumour Markers

K. D. Bagshawe

Cancer Research Campaign Laboratories, Department of Medical Oncology,
Charing Cross Hospital, London W6 8RF, United Kingdom

Introduction

The applications of tumour markers have widened in recent years. Initially they were seen to be a means of monitoring the course of the neoplastic process as a biochemical reflection of tumour cell burden. This remains their most important contemporary role although the difficulty of identifying such markers for the generality of cancers is well known. For a marker to have this function it must be secreted into body fluids where it can be detected, by some form of sensitive immunoassay. Such a marker may also have a diagnostic function provided it has the specificity to help discriminate between alternatives. Since the body burden of tumour is recognised to have a general correlation with prognosis a serum marker which reflects body burden can have the same significance as an estimation of tumour burden. Indeed it may provide a truer estimate of this than radiological methods.

A marker may have diagnostic or prognostic value in the context of immunocytochemistry and substances demonstrable by this technique are not necessarily secreted into body fluids. Further, it has become apparent that markers expressed in tumour cell membranes and not secreted into body fluids may have a special role in the new technique of radioimmunolocalisation and more speculatively as target molecules for antibody-directed therapeutic agents. These several roles for tumour markers mean that we need markers with different characteristics for different applications, and these fall into the broad categories of secreted and membrane-bound antigens respectively.

The possibility of finding completely specific markers for any form of human cancer has receded. Specificity is relative. What matters is whether a particular substance has, or may ultimately have, clinical utility. One may hope that organ-specific markers will be identified, but it is perhaps more realistic to think in terms of tissue-type-specific markers. Obviously, the ovary comprises several 'tissues' and at present there is no ovary-specific marker.

In contrast to the testis, where malignant germ cell tumours account for 90% of all neoplasms, in the ovary these account for only 1%–2% of all cancers. Good markers have been found for the germ cell tumours of both testis and ovary and, up to a point, these are models for what we need for the far commoner ovarian epithelial cancers.

For several years there has been much interest in the possibility of a good marker for ovarian epithelial cancer being defined and used as an aid to earlier diagnosis. There has been no shortage of contenders for this role. Many have been found and reported but have presumably failed to survive further evaluation. Studies of ovarian antigens not discussed further here include those reported by Levi (1971), Dorsett and Ioachim (1973),

Ovarian Cancer, Ed. by N. M. Bleehen

McGowan et al. (1973) and Gall et al. (1973). Nor shall I consider studies in cell-mediated immunology such as those of Hellstrom et al. (1971) and Pattillo et al. (1979), although it would, I think, be unwise to discount the potential value of this approach. Oestrogen and progesterone receptors have also been identified in ovarian carcinoma but again I do not propose to discuss these, although they have prognostic value (Spona et al. 1983).

It is probably right to view all new contenders for the marker role with some scepticism. Nevertheless, there are some grounds for supposing that useful, if not universal, markers for ovarian epithelial cancer may be emerging.

Markers for Ovarian Tumours

Alphafetoprotein (AFP)

There have been numerous reviews of alphafetoprotein in normal and tumour tissues (Abelev 1974; Bagshawe 1974; Thompson and Haddow 1979). The known sites of production of AFP in the fetus are yolk sac, liver and gastro-intestinal tract. In the adult there is a low serum level of AFP possibly from hepatic souces, although it is not readily demonstrated there. Hepatocellular carcinomas and yolk sac tumours (syn. endodermal sinus tumour, Teilum's tumour) produce it abundantly. Some germ cell tumours consist predominantly or exclusively of yolk sac elements. Others contain yolk sac elements but may also show additional components of a differentiated or undifferentiated nature.

AFP production reflects the activity only of the yolk sac component. The yolk sac component of the tumours of mixed histology may be readily identifiable morphologically but may be better demonstrated by immunocytochemistry. It should, however, be emphasised that substantial difficulty has been experienced in demonstrating AFP-producing cells by immunoperoxidase techniques on formalin-fixed tissues. No cells have yet been shown to produce both AFP and human chorionic gonadotrophin (HCG). We have found that about 75% of the germ cell tumours referred to us are associated with raised serum levels of AFP. There is no significant difference in the incidence of raised AFP levels between ovarian and testicular germ cell tumours.

AFP-producing germ cell tumours have been identified from birth onwards and it is clear that whenever such a tumour is a possibility AFP should be estimated. Tumours which are exclusively or predominantly yolk sac are found in prepubertal girls and serum AFP estimation can be used to aid diagnosis preoperatively.

In patients with germ cell tumours serum AFP measurements also have value as prognostic factors. We have found that patients with serum AFP > 500 kU/l had a worse prognosis than those with lower values, provided that HCG values were also taken into account. Serum AFP values undoubtedly reflect body burden of yolk sac tumour and may also reflect one of the most aggressive components in these tumours (Bagshawe and Begent 1983).

Monitoring AFP values provides a basis for graphical representation of the course of the yolk sac tumour. Computer graphics are a highly convenient way of presenting serial data from AFP and other markers in relation to therapeutic protocols; programs developed in our unit are now available commercially. The half-life of AFP is 4–6 days, so that clearance after complete surgical excision of a stage I tumour may seem slow. Persistence of AFP after this may be the only indication of metastatic disease, a state defined as stage I. M. In the course of chemotherapy the falling value of AFP indicates the response rate of the tumour. Failure of AFP values to fall may be the first indication of drug resistance.

Attention has recently been drawn to the fact that whereas the normal adult value for AFP rarely exceeds 3-10 kU/l and is usually <3 kU/l, patients receiving cis-platinum therapy may also show elevated values that sometimes exceed 50 kU/l (Coppack et al. 1983). The source of this AFP seems unlikely in all cases to be tumour, and may be of hepatic origin. Although differences in the concanavalin A binding characteristics of yolk sac and hepatic AFP have been identified it has not so far been possible to make this distinction at the low concentrations of AFP found in body fluids when this problem arises.

The technique of radioimmunolocalisation has been successfully used with AFP in several centres (Goldenberg et al. 1980; Begent and Bagshawe 1983).

Raised AFP values virtually exclude the presence of choriocarcinoma of gestational origin but both AFP and HCG are of course characteristic of many germ cell tumours as well as pregnancy.

Human Chorionic Gonadotrophin (HCG)

The role of HCG as a marker for gestational trophoblastic tumours including choriocarcinoma is well known and it is the nearest we get to the ideal secreted tumour marker (Bagshawe 1967, 1974; Seppala 1982). Just as AFP provides a marker for the yolk sac components of germ cell tumours so HCG reflects choriocarcinomatous elements (Fig. 1). A small percentage of germ cell tumours appear to be pure choriocarcinoma but more commonly there are other elements not reflected in HCG levels. In addition some dysgerminomas secrete HCG and this provides a valuable marker in such cases. Some tumours diagnosed morphologically as gonadoblastoma have also proved to produce HCG in amounts useful for clinical monitoring purposes.

In general, the amount of HCG reflects the burden of trophoblastic cells and reference has already been made to the prognostic effect of marker values (Bagshawe and Begent 1983). AFP and HCG appear to reflect the most aggressive elements in these tumours, so that when tumours of similar bulk are compared, those with higher AFP and HCG values carry a greater propensity for resistance to eradication by present methods.

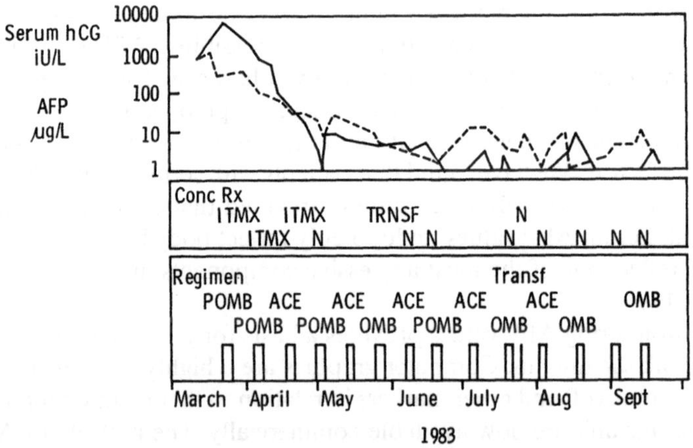

Fig. 1. Serum HCG and AFP values in management of patient with ovarian germ cell tumour. Conc Rx, concurrent therapy; ITMX, intrathecal methotrexate; N, diagnostic lumbar puncture normal; Transf, TRNSF, blood transfusion; POMB, cis-platinum, oncovin, methotrexate, bleomycin; ACE, actinomycin D, cyclophosphamide, etoposide

HCG production has been estimated to be of the order of 10^{-5} IU HCG per cell per day in choriocarcinoma. Its clearance rate is faster than that of AFP, the half-life being only 24–36 h. Rutanen and Seppala (1978) found that 18% of patients with ovarian cancers had detectable levels of HCG as did 14% of patients with non-malignant conditions. However, the extent to which these observations are related to high pituitary luteinising hormone (LH) values and cross-reaction between HCG and LH in the assay remains unclear. As assay technology continues to improve, this problem of cross-reactivity may be expected to be resolved, but it should be understood that the so-called β-HCG assays which are supposedly HCG specific, vary in their cross-reactivity. Also β-HCG assays usually detect both β-HCG and intact HCG, but intact HCG is the predominant form of the molecule. Although ectopic production of HCG or β-HCG by non-trophoblastic gynaecological tumours has been recognised the amount produced is small and it is uncommon for it to prove valuable in clinical monitoring. Alpha subunit has been identified in many studies in vitro but does not figure significantly as a useful marker in vivo in gynaecological tumours.

Pregnancy-Specific β-1-Glycoprotein (SP1)

SP1, like HCG, is a glycoprotein produced by syncytiotrophoblast (Bohn 1971). Generally the serum concentration is lower than that of HCG, although exceptions have been reported (Seppala et al. 1978). Marginally raised values have been recorded in non-trophoblastic gynaecological tumours (Wurz 1979; Crowther et al. 1979) but the clinical value of such measurements has not been demonstrated.

PP5

A whole series of placental proteins, PP_2–PP_{14}, have been defined by Bohn and his colleagues (Bohn and Winkler 1977). PP_5 is a syncytiotrophoblastic product. It has not so far been demonstrated to have a role in clinical oncology although ectopic production has been recorded.

Placental Alkaline Phosphatase (PLAP)

Placental type alkaline phosphatase is characterised by being heat stable and L-phenylalanine sensitive and was first identified by enzymic assay in ovarian and other tumours by Fishman et al. (1968). PLAP and a closely related variant, Regan isoenzyme, have been found in various tumours. An L-leucine sensitive form is known as the Nagao isoenzyme; the Kasahara isoenzyme corresponds to fetal intestinal alkaline phosphatase. These also have been found in tumours and may be present in ascitic fluid of ovarian carcinomas (reviewed by Fishman 1983).

Rarely a tumour has been found to produce large amounts of PLAP, but mostly only small amounts are secreted. This is true even of trophoblastic tumours where it is produced by syncytium and possibly to a much lesser extent by cytotrophoblast. It has, however, been demonstrated in both benign and malignant ovarian tumours (Benham et al. 1978).

Its main interest as a serum marker lies in its value in some cases of germinoma (Wah-

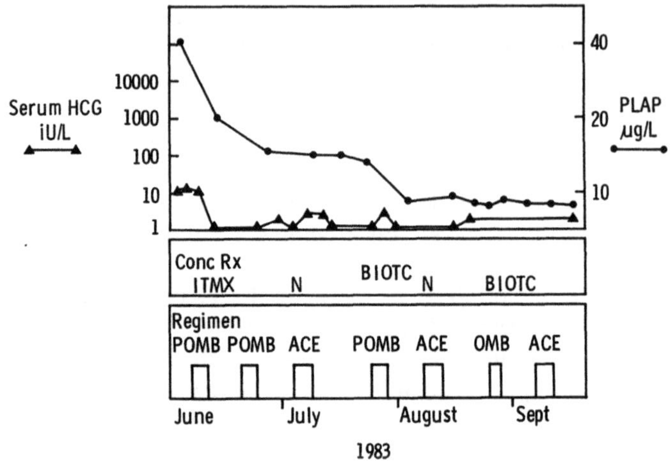

Fig. 2. Serum placental alkaline phosphatase (PLAP) and human chorionic gonadotrophin (HCG) in a patient with germ cell tumour and germinoma elements. Abbreviations as in Fig. 1; BIOTC, antibiotic therapy

Table 1. Serum placental alkaline phosphatase values (> 8 ng/ml)

Miscellaneous malignancies	3/6
Mixed germ cell tumours of testis	22/33
Seminoma	
Stage I	21/37
Stage II	10/14
Malignant teratoma of testis	14/57
Ovarian epithelial cancer	13/35
Ascitic fluid with ovarian cancer	6/12
Normal subjects	1/52
Patients with non-malignant disease	6/119
Chronic renal failure	8/48

ren et al. 1979; Lange et al. 1982). It requires further investigation in ovarian epithelial cancer, where studies show that about a third of patients have raised values.

It is also of interest as a membrane marker for other germ cell tumours, where it may provide a serum marker (Fig. 2) or be used for radioimmunolocalsation and perhaps for drug targeting. Our own preliminary studies have also identified PLAP in a high proportion of cells in malignant epithelial ovarian tumours and in some patients' sera. (Table 1). Detailed immunocytochemical studies of its distribution are in progress. The development of a series of monoclonal antibodies for PLAP has provided an interesting tool for the evaluation of this complex group of isoenzymes as well as a basis for immunoassays, radioimmunolocalisation and possibly drug targeting.

Lactic Dehydrogenase (LDH)

LDH is a glycolytic enzyme present in various tissues and existing as at least five different isoenzymes. Elevated levels have been noted in the serum of patients with various cancers and leukaemias (Hill and Levi 1954).

It appears to be a useful marker in some patients with germ cell tumours (von Eyben 1978), including dysgerminomas, where the fast fraction appears to be derived from the germinoma cells. Elevated values may be found in those patients in the presence of normal AFP and HCG (Fig. 2). Relapse has been first indicated by rising LDH values in some patients (Sheiko and Hart 1982).

Elevated values have also been reported in the serum of patients with ovarian adenocarcinomas; however it is not clear from reports whether the values are more than marginally elevated.

Ferritin

Ferritin is not a tumour product but has been proposed as an additional marker for germ cell tumours. In particular it is suggested that persistently elevated serum ferritin may have prognostic value (Grail et al. 1982). More detailed studies in parallel with those on other markers are needed for a full evaluation.

Galactosyltransferase (Lactose Synthase, GTT)

Reports that the galactosyltransferase activity in ovarian tumour homogenates was higher than in normal ovary (Bhattacharya et al. 1976) have been followed by further evidence that this enzyme may be a useful marker (Chatterjee et al. 1979). Although it may also be produced in excess by hepatic tissue there is evidence that it is produced by tumour cells. The existing enzymic assays have not proved convenient and the development of immunoassays has been impeded by difficulties in raising specific antibodies.

Verdon et al. (1983) have recently reported the use of an enzyme-linked immunosorbent assay (ELISA) giving values of 60–436 μg/l in normal subjects. In small groups of patients with ovarian, breast and lung cancer values were found in the range 129–1156 μg/l. In ovarian cancer the GTT level appeared to reflect tumour burden.

OCAA

An ovarian cystadenocarcinoma-associated antigen (OCAA) was found by Bhattachaarya and Barlow (1975) to be present in all serous adenocarcinomas and cystadenocarcinomas of the ovary. A second antigen was defined by these workers as OCAA1 and this has been identified in serum (for review see Bagshawe et al. 1979).

OCA

OCA, an antigen described by Knauf and Urbach (1978), showed some cross-reactivity with carcinoembryonic antigen (CEA) but was distinct from it on several criteria. In patients with ovarian tumours it was found to be more sensitive than CEA. Its clinical usefulness does not appear to have been established at the present time.

OvC-1 and OvC-6

A series of antigens from human ovarian cancer have been isolated by Imamura et al. (1978). Some were related to CEA and cross-reacting antigens.

6K Peptide

A urinary peptide of molecular weight 6000 has been characterised by Stenman et al. (1982). Elevated values in urine were reported in 5/8 patients with ovarian cancer, 10/14 with carcinoma of the cervix and 9/14 with endometrial cancer.

Carcinoembryonic Antigen (CEA)

The contribution of CEA, a widely used marker in patients with ovarian cancer, has been rather disappointing. Although there may be molecular heterogeneity and different assay systems may give different numerical values for CEA concentrations, no particular assay or antibody has proved significantly superior overall. CEA in gynaecological tumours has not been proved to be distinguishable from that associated with colonic carcinoma. Some workers have found raised CEA levels in over 75% of patients with ovarian cancer (Khoo and Mackay 1976) but others have found a much lower incidence (Stone et al. 1977; Seppala 1982). In general the degree of elevation has been modest and then it has only been detected in disease of relatively advanced stage. The fact that many groups of workers have continued to seek better markers for ovarian cancer indicates the inadequacies of CEA as a serum marker.

As a marker for radioimmunolocalisation it may have a place, although it may be speculated that other markers such as PLAP will prove superior.

CX1

CX1 is a glycoprotein, first described by Wass et al. (1981) and formerly designated OTAG. It was isolated from an ovarian serous cystadenocarcinoma and subsequently identified in the serum and ascitic fluids of patients with ovarian epithelial cancers. It also proved to be detectable at concentrations of up to 70 μg/l in normal sera. It has been found to be present in increased concentration in about 60% of patients with stage III or IV ovarian adenocarcinoma and in the sera of patients with other advanced carcinomas. Its concentration appears to reflect tumour burden. However, the low detection rate in stage II and in clinical remission has proved to be a limitation, and although it is a useful marker in some patients it is less reliable than is desirable for clinical purposes. Lead-in times in relapse after therapy have ranged from zero up to 4 months.

CA 19-9

CA 19-9 is a carbohydrate determinant that has been defined by monoclonal antibody methods (Koprowski et al. 1979) and is known to be distributed in a range of tumours. Assay kits have become available. In one immunocytochemical study a high proportion of mucinous adenocarcinomas gave positive results, as did a lower proportion of serous adenocarcinomas. As a serum marker for ovarian cancer it appears to add little to CEA values, but more data are needed for a full evaluation.

CA 125

The monoclonal antibody OC 125 was raised by immunisation with an ovarian epithelial cell line OVCA433 (Bast et al. 1981). The antigen detected by this antibody has been designated CA 125, and is associated with a high-molecular-weight glycoprotein expressed in fetal coelomic epithelium. It has not been identified in normal ovarian tissue. It is a secreted antigen and a radioimmunometric assay has recently been reported.

Taking an upper normal value of 35 μg/ml, only 1% of 888 healthy individuals and 6% of 143 patients with non-malignant disease had elevated values, compared with 83 of 101 patients with ovarian epithelial cancer. Rising and falling values were found to correlate with the course of the disease in 93% of cases and values ranged up to 8000 U/ml (Bast et al. 1983). Elevated values were also found in 12%–59% of patients with carcinomas of the pancreas, colon, rectum, lung, breast etc., but most of these had values that did not exceed 65 U/ml. If an upper normal value of 65 U/ml is taken, then the percentage of ovarian cancer patients with raised values falls to about 70%, but clearly the staging of cases in relation to positivity is important in this regard and few data are so far available. A lead-in time from rising values to clinical relapse of 7 months was reported in one case.

On published evidence this would appear to be the most promising of the markers so far detected in the serum of ovarian cancer patients. It is already available in the form of a commercial kit and the question that will inevitably arise in cost-conscious countries is whether its potential contribution to clinical management and to patient survival justifies the cost.

791T/36

One of the recurring features of work in the field of tumour markers is the finding that antibodies evoked by immunisation with one form of cancer may react with tumours of seemingly unrelated tissues. Price et al. (1983) reported the characteristics of a monoclonal antibody raised to osteosarcoma cells. Later it was reported also to localise in ovarian epithelial cancers. The antigen, 791T/36, is associated with cell membranes and it is not yet known whether it is secreted into serum in significant amounts. It has, however, been used successfully in the technique of radioimmunolocalisation in some patients with ovarian cancer.

Discussion

The practical contribution of these efforts to improve the management of ovarian cancer has so far been small, with the exception of the germ cell tumours where by contrast the contribution of tumour markers is substantial. It may be a coincidence that the prognosis of patients with advanced germ cell tumours has changed dramatically from near zero to better than 75% long-term survival and that the prognosis for patients with the epithelial tumours has changed little. Nevertheless it would be unwise to underestimate the contribution which a good tumour marker can make, though clearly a marker does not of itself substitute for effective therapy and its value may only become apparent when good therapy appears on the scene. We have, of course, the enticing prospect that good markers may provide the homing beacons for antibody-directed therapy, but it would be easy to underestimate the formidable obstacles that remain to this approach.

What is moderately encouraging in the area of ovarian epithelial cancer is that a number of secreted markers appear capable of making some contribution to clinical management and collectively perhaps their individual contributions may be enhanced. On present evidence CA 125 is the most promising serum marker and it remains to be determined whether this conclusion is substantiated in the hard light of practice and whether CX1, CEA and possibly CA 19-9 add anything useful.

CX1, CA 125 and PLAP have been used as aids in the diagnosis of ascites due to ovarian cancer, although specificity cannot be sufficient to exclude other neoplastic causes. The membrane-bound antigens may also need further evaluation here, although it is not common for such ascites to constitute a major diagnostic hurdle. The critical test for the membrane-bound marker is the proportion of tumour cells, and more specifically, of clonogenic cells, in the tumour that express the antigen. It is this that will determine a marker's potential for drug targeting. Given that present methods of therapy rarely eliminate advanced ovarian adenocarcinoma, a good marker would still detect residual disease in these patients in clinical remmission. We have some way to go before that goal is reached.

References

Abelev GI (1974) Alphafetoprotein as a marker of embryo-specific differentiations in normal and tumour tissues. Transplant Rev 20: 3-37

Bagshawe KD (1967) Comments on the measurement of HCG as a tumour specific substance. In: JA Holland, MM Hreshchyshyn (eds) Choriocarcinoma. UICC Monograph Series 3. Springer-Verlag, Berlin Heidelberg New York, pp 109-111

Bagshawe KD (1974) Tumour associated antigens. Br Med Bull 30: 68-73

Bagshawe KD, Begent RHJ (1983) Staging, markers and prognostic factors. In: KD Bagshawe, RHJ Begent, ES Newlands (eds) Germ cell tumours. Clinics in oncology. W.B. Saunders, London, pp 159-181

Bagshawe KD, Wass M, Searle F (1979) Glycoproteins in ovarian cancer. In: E Boelsma, PH Rumke (eds) Tumour markers. Elsevier Solidus North-Holland Biomedical Press, Amsterdam, pp 79-87

Bast RC Jr, Feeney M, Lazarus H, Nadler LM, Colvin RB, Knapp RC (1981) Reactivity of a monoclonal antibody with human ovarian carcinoma. J Clin Invest 68: 1331-1337

Bast RC Jr, Klug TL, St John E, Knapp RC (1983) A radioimmunoassay using a monoclonal antibody to monitor the course of epithelial ovarian cancer. N Engl J Med 309: 883-887

Begent RH, Bagshawe KD (1983) Radioimmunolocalisation of cancer. In: Fishman WH (ed) Oncodevelopmental markers. Academic Press, New York London, pp 167-188

Benham FJ, Povey MS, Harris H (1978) Placental-like alkaline phosphatase in malignant and benign ovarian tumours. Clin Chim Acta 86: 201-215

Bhattacharya M, Barlow JJ (1975) Tumour associated antigen for cystadenocarcinomas of the ovary. Natl Cancer Inst Monogr 42: 25-32

Bhattacharya M, Chatterjee SK, Barlow JJ (1976) Uridine 5-diphosphate galactose: glycoprotein galactosyl transferase activity in the ovarian cancer patient. Cancer Res 36: 2096-2101

Bohn H (1971) Nachweis und Charakterisierung von Schwangerschaftsproteinen in der menschlichen Placenta. Arch Gynaekol 210: 440-457

Bohn H, Winkler W (1977) Isolierung und Charakterisierung des Plazenta-Proteins PP_5. Arch Gynaekol 223: 179-186
Chatterjee SK, Bhattacharya M, Barlow JL (1979) Glycosyltransferase and glycosidase activities in ovarian cancer patients. Cancer Res 39: 1943-1951
Coppack S, Newlands ES, Dent J, Mitchell H, Goka G, Bagshawe KD (1983) Problems of interpretation of serum concentration of alphafetoprotein in patients receiving cytotoxic chemotherapy for malignant germ cell tumours. Br J Cancer 48: 335-340
Crowther ME, Grundzinkas JG, Poulton JA, Gordon YB (1979) Trophoblastic proteins in ovarian carcinoma. Obstet Gynecol 53: 59-61
Dorsett BH, Ioachim HL (1973) Common antigenic component in ovarian carcinomas: Demonstration by double diffusion and immunofluorescence techniques. Immunol Comm 2: 173-184
Fishman WH (1983) Oncodevelopmental markers. In: WH Fishman (ed) Oncodevelopmental markers. Academic Press, New York London, pp 3-19
Fishman WH, Inglis NR, Stolbach LL, Krant MJA (1968) Serum alkaline phosphatase isoenzyme of human neoplastic cell origin. Cancer Res 28: 150-154
Gall SA, Walling J, Pearl J (1973) Demonstration of tumour associated antigens in human gynecologic malignancy. Am J Obstet Gynecol 115: 387-393
Goldenberg DM, Kim E, Deland E, Spremulli E, Nelson JP, Primus FJ, Alpert E (1980) Clinical studies in the radioimmunodetection of tumours containing alpha-fetoprotein. Cancer 45: 2500-2505
Grail A, Bates G, Milford Ward A, Jones WG, Hancock BW (1982) Serum ferritin as a third marker in germ cell tumours. Eur J Cancer Clin Oncol 18: 261-269
Hellstrom I, Hellstrom KE, Sjogren HO, Warner GA (1971) Demonstration of cell-mediated immunity to human neoplasms of various histological types. Int J Cancer 7: 1-16
Hill BR, Levi C (1954) Elevation of serum component in neoplastic disease. Cancer Res 14: 513-515
Imamura N, Takahashi T, Lloyd KO, Lewis JL, Old LJ (1978) Analysis of human ovarian tumour antigens using heterologous antisera: Detection of new antigenic systems. Int J Cancer 21: 570-577
Khoo SK, Mackay EV (1976) Carcinoembryonic antigen (CEA) in ovarian cancer. Factors affecting its incidence and changes which occur in response to cytotoxic drugs. Br J Obstet Gynaecol 83: 753-759
Knauf S, Urbach GI (1978) The development of a double antibody radioimmunoassay for detecting ovarian tumour associated antigen fraction OCA in plasma. Am J Obstet Gynecol 131: 780-787
Koprowski H, Steplewski Z, Mitchell K, Herlyn M, Herlyn D, Fuhrer P (1979) Colorectal carcinoma antigens detected by hybridoma antibodies. Somatic Cell Genet 5: 957-971
Lange PH, Millan JL, Stigbrand T, Vessella RL, Ruoslahti E, Fishman WH (1982) Placental alkaline phosphatase as a tumour marker for seminoma. Cancer Res 42: 3244-3247
Levi MM (1971) Antigenicity of ovarian and cervical malignancies with a view to possible immunodiagnosis. Am J Obstet Gynecol 109: 689-698
McGowan L, Davis RH, Bunnag B (1973) The biochemical diagnosis of ovarian cancer. Am J Obstet Gynecol 116: 760-768
Pattillo RA, Ruckert ACF, Story MT, Mattingly RF (1979) Immunodiagnosis in ovarian cancer. Am J Obstet Gynecol 133: 791-799
Price MR, Campbell DG, Robins RA, Baldwin RW (1983) Characteristics of a cell surface antigen defined by an anti-human osteogenic sarcoma monoclonal antibody. Eur J Cancer 19: 81-90
Rutanen EM, Seppala M (1978) The HCG-beta subunit radioimmunoassay in non-trophoblastic gynaecologic tumours. Cancer 41: 692-696
Seppala M (1982) Ovarian and uterine cancer markers. In: S Sell, B Wahren (eds) Human cancer markers. Humana Press, Clifton, New Jersey, pp 233-257
Seppala M, Rutanen EM, Heikinheimo M, Jalanko H, Engvall E (1978) Detection of trophoblastic tumour activity Int J Cancer 21: 265-267
Sheiko MC, Hart WP (1982) Ovarian germinoma (dysgerminoma) with elevated serum lactic dehydrogenase. Cancer 49: 994-998

Spona J, Gitsch E, Salzer H, Karrer K (1983) Estrogen and gestagen receptors in ovarian carcinoma. Gynecol Obstet Invest 16: 189-198

Stenman U, Huhtala M-L, Koistinen R, Seppala M (1982) Immunochemical demonstration of an ovarian cancer associated urinary peptide. Int J Cancer 30: 53-57

Stone M, Bagshawe KD, Kardana A, Searle F, Dent J (1977) Beta-human chorionic gonadotrophin and carcinoembryonic antigen in the management of ovarian carcinoma. Br J Obstet Gynaecol 84: 375-379

Thompson DK, Haddow Je (1979) Serial monitoring of serum alphafetoprotein and chorionic gonadotrophin in males with germ cell tumours. Cancer 43: 1820-1829

Verdon B, Berger EG, Salehli S, Goldhirsch A, Gerber A (1983) An enzyme linked immunosorbent assay for lactose synthase (galactosyltransferase) in serum and its application as a tumour marker in ovarian carcinoma. Clin Chem 29: 1928-1933

von Eyben FE (1978) Biochemical markers in advanced testicular tumours. Cancer 41: 648-652

Wahren B, Holmgren PA, Stigbrand T (1979) Placental alkaline phosphatase, alphafetoprotein and carcinoembryonic antigen in testicular tumours. Tissue typing by means of cytologic smears. Int J Cancer 24: 749-753

Wass M, Searle F, Bagshawe KD (1981) Radioimmunoassay of the normal serum glycoprotein (CX1) in monitoring ovarian malignancy. Eur J Cancer Clin Oncol 17: 1267-1273

Wurz H (1979) Serum concentrations of SP_1 in healthy non-pregnant individuals and in patients with non-trophoblastic neoplasms. Arch Gynaekol 227: 1-6

X-Ray Techniques and Ultrasound in Diagnosis and Staging

R. J. Johnson*

Department of Diagnostic Radiology, University of Manchester, and Christie Hospital and Holt Radium Institute, Manchester M20 9BX, United Kingdom

Introduction

Carcinoma of the ovary is the commonest cause of death from gynaecological malignancy in the United Kingdom and United States, accounting for approximately 3500 deaths per annum in England and Wales (OPCS Mortality Statistics 1982) and 11000 deaths per annum in the United States (Cancer Facts and Figures 1975). Five-year survival figures related to the stage of disease at presentation are detailed in Table 1. The overall 5 year survival has not improved significantly in the past few decades, rising in the United States from 29% during the period 1950-59 to 32% during the period 1965-69 (Cutler et al. 1975). This poor survival is related in part to the fact that only 30% of patients have localised tumour at the time of diagnosis (Julian and Woodruff 1969), the majority of patients presenting with Stage III and IV disease (Day and Smith 1975; Fisher and Young 1977; Watring et al. 1979).

The early detection of asymptomatic ovarian carcinoma and advances in treatment for extensive disease may improve the survival figures. Between 20% and 50% of women who have received surgery with or without additional radiotherapy for localised disease (Stage I and II) will relapse and require further treatment (Munnel 1968; Bagley et al. 1972). Some of these patients will have been understaged at initial diagnosis (Bagley et al.

Table 1. Relation of stage to prognosis

Stage	No. of patients	5-year survival (%)
I	751	61
IA	528	65
IB	130	52
IC	80	52
II	401	40
IIA	40	60
IIB	205	38
III	539	5
IV	101	3

Taken from Tobias and Griffiths (1976). N Engl J Med 294: 818-823. Based on data of Parker et al., Van Orden et al., Sall and Stone, Kottmeier, Kent, McKay and Aure et al. (comprising 1792 patients)

* I would like to thank my clinical colleagues for their help and advice, Mrs Lang for typing the manuscript and Mr Griffin for preparing the illustrations

Ovarian Cancer, Ed. by N. M. Bleehen

1973; Knapp and Friedman 1974; Rosenoff et al. 1975). Accurate staging, enabling optimal treatment, may prevent relapse and further improve the survival figures.

Radiology has been of limited value in the clinical management of ovarian carcinoma. The introduction of lymphography and the non-invasive techniques of ultrasound (US) and computerised tomography (CT) has increased the potential role of radiology in the diagnosis, staging and assessment of therapy in ovarian carcinoma. In this review attention will be focused on these techniques. The role of US and CT scanning in the diagnosis of a pelvic mass is discussed in the first section, as is the role of US in the early diagnosis of ovarian carcinoma. In the second section the use of CT and US scanning and lymphography in the staging of ovarian carcinoma is described. Radionuclide imaging is discussed in the following chapter.

The Role of Radiology in Diagnosis of Ovarian Carcinoma

Symptoms of early ovarian carcinoma are uncommon. The tumour grows insidiously with 60%-70% of patients presenting with stage III and IV disease. The patients have non-specific abdominal pain or discomfort, increasing abdominal girth from the tumour bulk or ascites and a palpable mass. Clinicians often proceed to laparotomy in these cases with minimal radiological investigations. Such investigations include a chest radiograph, an intravenous urogram (IVU) and occasionally barium studies. The chest radiograph will demonstrate the presence of any pleural effusion of more than 600 ml, and the IVU delineates the anatomy of the renal tract, in particular the number and course of the ureters and the presence of any ureteric obstruction. A barium enema will identify those patients who require bowel resection or diversion.

The 30% of patients who present with localised disease usually have a palpable mass found on routine examination or as an incidental finding at surgery for non-related disease (Fisher and Young 1977). The finding of a pelvic mass in a female of any age can cause problems in diagnosis and management. Increasing emphasis is placed on radiology in these situations and the methods available are detailed in Table 2.

The value and role of the various imaging techniques must be seen in relation to current clinical practice. At present it is accepted that all prepubertal, perimenopausal and postmenopausal women with a palpable adnexal mass greater than 5-6 cm in diameter should have an exploratory operation to exclude or confirm the diagnosis of ovarian carcinoma (Day and Smith 1975; Watring et al. 1979). Barber and Graber (1971) have suggested that a palpable ovary in the postmenopausal woman is abnormal and that these patients should undergo surgery to improve the early detection of ovarian carcinoma. Adnexal masses detected in women during the reproductive years can be observed for a period of time, usually to a similar time in the next menstrual cycle, if they are cystic and less

Table 2. Techniques for imaging a pelvic mass

Indirect	*Direct*
Plain abdomino-pelvic radiograph	Ultrasound (US)
Intravenous urogram (IVU)	Computerised tomography (CT)
Barium studies	Arteriography and venography
	Magnetic resonance (NMR)

than 5 cm in diameter. Masses larger than 5-6 cm, in diameter may require surgical removal to prevent torsion or rupture and to exclude malignancy (Schwartz and Weiner 1979). Experienced clinicians who identify and adnexal mass usually feel that radiological investigation is superfluous (Schwartz and Weiner 1979) as management is based on the history and pelvic examination. However, radiology is important when the site of origin of the mass cannot be determined clinically or when the pelvic examination is inadequate. This may occur in children, obese patients or those who have undergone previous surgery or pelvic radiotherapy. Persistent pelvic pain with a negative clinical examination is an indication for further investigation and even in those patients where the surgeon is confident of his findings and proposed management radiological investigations may identify unsuspected pathology.

Imaging Techniques

Plain radiographs, intravenous urography (IVU) and barium studies are of limited value in assessing a pelvic mass. The abdomino-pelvic radiograph may reveal a soft tissue mass displacing the bowel or the presence of calcification. The amorphous calcification of a uterine fibroid can usually be differentiated from the psammomatous calcification of ovarian malignancy, which occurs in approximately 12% of patients with serous cystadenoma or serous cystadenocarcinoma (Lewis et al. 1982). Masses containing fat and calcific density, often with dental elements, are diagnostic of an ovarian teratoma or dermoid. The IVU provides little diagnostic information but is important in defining the course of the ureters and identifying pelvic kidneys. A barium enema will identify primary colorectal carcinoma which can present as a pelvic mass simulating ovarian malignancy and will also demonstrate secondary bowel involvement by ovarian carcinoma. Arteriography and venography have been largely superseded by ultrasound and computerised tomography.

Ultrasound (US)

The development and refinement of US techniques over the past 20 years has resulted in their increasing use in clinical practice. The female pelvis is usually examined by a transabdominal technique using the distended bladder as an acoustic window. Conventional grey-scale B mode and real-time equipment is used. The procedure is non-invasive and is acceptable to the majority of patients. Fluid-filled loops of bowel can simulate pelvic masses but the use of real-time equipment should demonstrate a change in configuration of the mass due to peristalsis. Modern equipment can resolve cystic lesions in the order of 1-2 cm in diameter, and solid lesions 2-3 cm in diameter.

The accuracy of US in the detection and localisation of a pelvic mass is in the order of 90% when compared with surgical findings (Levi and Delval 1976; Lawson and Albarelli 1977; Fleisher et al. 1978; Walsh et al. 1979; DeLand et al. 1979). Reliable information can also be obtained about the size and consistency of the mass and criteria for the distinction of benign from malignant ovarian cysts have been reported (Morley and Barnett 1970; Meire et al. 1978). Benign lesions are usually unilocular cysts of if multilocular have thin septa (<3 mm). No nodules are present. Malignant lesions are usually multilocular with thin septa and nodules present or they have thick septa (>3 mm) with or without nodules. Meire et al. (1978) claim a 91% accuracy in distinguishing benign from malignant lesions using these criteria.

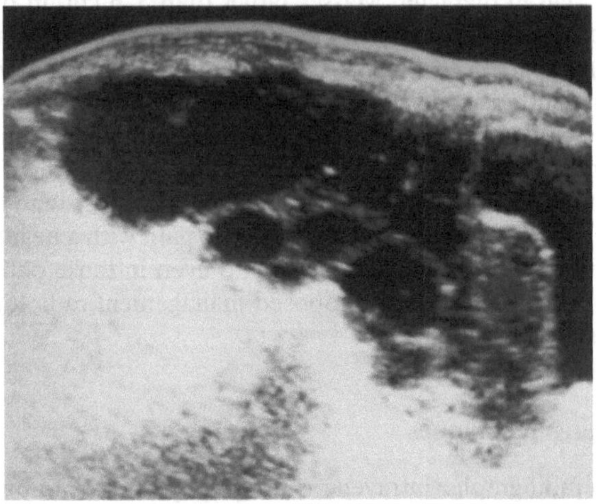

Fig. 1. Sagittal US scan demonstrating an enlarged uterus which is pressing on the bladder. Within the uterus is an area of increased echo amplitude due to calcification within a uterine fibroid

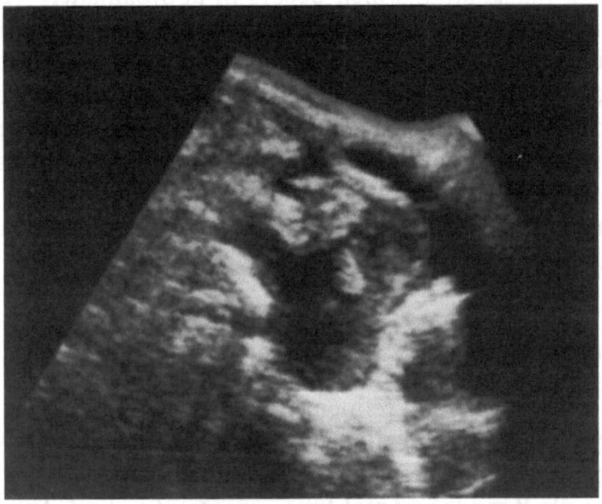

Fig. 2. Sagittal US scan demonstrating a multilocular cystic mass with thick septa and nodules. The appearances are those of an adenoid cystic ovarian carcinoma.

An analysis of all the findings will indicate the probable diagnosis (Fig. 1 and 2) or provide a short-list of differential diagnoses. Kobayashi (1976) reported a greater than 70% accuracy in distinguishing carcinoma of the ovary from other types of malignant pelvic tumours and DeLand et al. (1979) were able to differentiate ovarian tumours from other pelvic tumours in more than 90% of their patients. Walsh et al. (1979) made a correct diagnosis in 56% of 204 patients with a pelvic mass. They felt a specific histological diagnosis was possible in selected patients with simple ovarian cysts, cystadenomas, cystadenocarcinomas, dermoid tumours and other non-ovarian lesions. However, the criteria used to make specific diagnoses may be unreliable (Requard et al. 1981; Moyle et al. 1983). US is not able to characterise tissue; the appearances seen on the scan reflect the morphology of the lesion and not its histology.

Computerised Tomography (CT)

Computerised tomography, whilst a non-invasive technique, employs ionising radiation and is less available than US to the majority of clinicians, particularly in the United Kingdom. In the assessment of patients with a pelvic mass CT will provide similar information to US (Walsh et al. 1978; Amendola et al. 1981; Coulam et al. 1982). Sanders et al. (1983) in a prospective study of CT and US in the detection and staging of pelvic masses found no significant difference in the ability of the two modalities to identify the mass or to predict the extent of disease. The sensitivities of CT and US in the detection of a pelvic mass were 0.96 and 0.91 respectively. The criteria for diagnosis of an ovarian lesion and deciding whether it is benign or malignant are similar to those used in US. However, like US, CT cannot characterise tissue and the histological type of tumour cannot be predicted.

"Walsh et al. (1978) state that ultrasound will identify the ovarian origin of a pelvic mass more consistently than CT, and in two out of nine patients in the series of Amendola et al. (1981) who had a pre operative CT scan, and ovarian mass could not be distinguished from the uterus. Coulam et al. (1982) thought US was the technique of choice for the initial evaluation of a cystic ovarian tumour."

US and CT Guided-Needle Biopsy

The introduction of percutaneous guided-needle biopsy techniques enables specimens to be obtained for tissue diagnosis from lesions in the abdomen and pelvis. This can be helpful in patients with an ovarian mass who have a known primary elsewhere. Cytological examination may distinguish whether the lesion is a metastasis or a second primary, and thereby affect patient management. The techniques can be adapted for the aspiration and drainage of fluid collections within the pelvis or abdomen.

Magnetic Resonance Imaging

Nuclear magnetic resonance (NMR) is a new technique of imaging. Like CT and US scanning it is non-invasive but unlike CT does not use ionising radiation and is capable of imaging directly in the transverse axial, coronal and sagittal planes. The pelvis is ideally suited to NMR imaging because of the natural contrast provided by fat, urine in the bladder and bowel gas. This natural contrast together with multi-planar imaging makes NMR a promising technique for staging pelvic malignancies. More important is the potential for tissue characterisation and the ability to distinguish between benign and malignant lesions. Initital experiences of NMR scanning in the pelvis have been reported (Bryan et al. 1983; Hricak et al. 1983). Fig. 3 demonstrates the appearance of an ovarian tumour obtained using a 0.26 tesla superconductive magnet.

Summary

Indirect imaging techniques are of limited value in the radiological assessment of a pelvic mass. The direct imaging techniques of US and CT provide more useful information and pointers to the diagnosis. Although US is more operator dependent than CT it has some

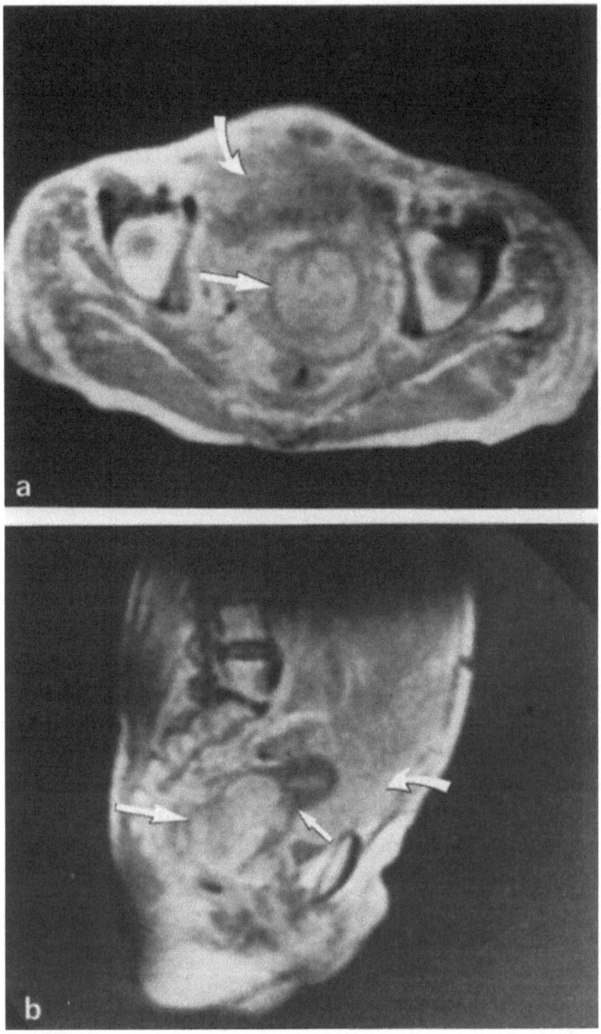

Fig. 3 a, b. MR Image Ovarian carcinoma. Spin echo (TR = 1000 ms, TE = 60 ms) images in the transverse axial (a) and parasagittal planes (b) demonstrate the cystic tumour (large straight arrow) and ascites (curved arrow). On the parasagittal image the tumour is seen to involve the uterus (small straight arrow)

advantages over the latter which make it the investigation of choice in those situations described above when clinicians require more information than can be obtained by pelvic examination. The advantages of US over CT are:

1. It is more widely available and cheaper.
2. It does not use ionising radiation.
3. It requires less patient preparation.
4. It appears to have a slight superiority over CT in detecting ovarian lesions.
5. It can image the normal ovary.

If the US examination is technically difficult or the result equivocal then a pelvic CT scan is justified.

Percutaneous needle biopsy techniques under US guidance are useful in certain situations to obtain specimens for tissue diagnosis. NMR is a promising technique for characterising pelvic masses and staging pelvic malignancy.

The Early Diagnosis of Ovarian Carcinoma

Ovarian carcinoma is usually asymptomatic in the early stages and detection will remain a chance occurrence unless a reliable screening test is found. Routine annual pelvic examinations and cervical cytology have not improved the detection rate (Tobias and Griffiths 1976). Examination of peritoneal fluid by transvaginal aspiration is impracticable for routine use (McGowan et al. 1966; Julian and Woodruff 1969).

The identification of a specific tumour marker would be ideal. A monoclonal antibody (OC 125) has been developed which reacts with a cell-surface antigen on epithelial ovarian tumour cells (Kabawat et al. 1983). This antigen, designated CA 125, has been detected in sera from patients with epithelial ovarian carcinoma (Bast et al. 1983) and may be a clinically useful tumour marker.

Ultrasound may provide an accurate screening method. Modern grey-scale equipment can identify cystic lesions less than 1 cm in diameter that are undetectable clinically (Meire et al. 1978). Although little is documented about the initial morphological change in ovarian carcinoma, 94% will develop cystic spaces (McGowan 1978). Campbell et al. (1982) recently obtained reliable measurements of ovarian volume in postmenopausal women using real-time equipment and also identified changes in ovarian morphology. They believe that an ovary with a volume twice that of the calculated mean or twice the size of the opposite ovary should be regarded with suspicion. It is known that the ovary decreases in size in the menopausal woman and Barber and Graber (1971) have previously advocated that postmenopausal women with a palpable ovary should undergo laparotomy.

Whilst cost and shortage of manpower may be objections to the use of US as a screening procedure, a prospective study comparing US findings with clinical examination and surgery is warranted.

Radiological Techniques in the Staging of Ovarian Carcinoma

The International Federation of Gynaecology and Obstetrics (FIGO) staging system is based on the concept that ovarian cancer spreads first within the pelvis, then within the peritoneum and does not metastasise outside the peritoneum until quite late in the course of the disease. Five pathways of metastatic spread have been described:

1. Local extension to contiguous structures.
2. Transcoelomic spread to involve the peritoneum including the undersurface of the hemi-diaphragms, liver capsule, omentum and visceral serosa.
3. Lymphatic spread to involve iliac, para-aortic and paracaval nodes.
4. Haematogenous spread to the liver parenchyma and rarely to lung or bone.
5. Transdiaphragmatic lymphatic spread to involve mediastinal nodes.

The inability of radiological techniques to characterise tissue and to detect lesions less than 1 cm in diameter prevents them from replacing surgery as a staging investigation.

Histological samples need to be obtained and often the only evidence of spread of disease at the time of surgery is the presence of peritoneal seedlings less than 0.5 cm in diameter. These would not be detected radiologically. Also the initial abdominal exploration and surgical procedures undertaken have a greater bearing on survival than any subsequent therapy (Tobias and Griffiths 1976).

As most patients will undergo surgery, the extent to which radiological techniques are used as staging procedures pre-operatively varies from centre to centre. In women with a palpable mass who have been referred for pelvic US or CT examination the identification of an ovarian lesion with features of malignancy may justify examination of the abdomen. Special attention will need to be given to the predicted sites of metastatic spread (Marglin and Castellino 1981). The role of pre-operative lymphography is controversial. Some centres untertake the investigation routinely (Musumeci et al. 1980). Watring et al. (1979) advocate the use of lymphography combined with guided-needle biopsy of suspicious nodes when abdominal exploration is not planned. However, it does not seem necessary to undertake this procedure in those patients with clinical stage III and IV disease as it will not alter the immediate management. Whilst it is important to document disease outside the pelvis in patients with clinical stage I and II disease there must be few circumstances in which abdominal exploration would not be undertaken. Lymphography is a minor surgical procedure and time-conumsing, and although complications are infrequent it is difficult to justify its routine pre-operative use in patients in whom a diagnosis of malignancy is not proven and who may have a benign lesion.

The major role of radiological staging is after the initial surgery and in the follow-up period when CT, US and lymphography are used:

1. As an adjunct to surgical staging.
2. To obtain baseline measurements of post-operative residual disease before further surgery.
3. To re-stage the patients following therapy and evaluate tumour response by measuring volume change.
4. As a guide to second-look laparotomy.

The value of these techniques is discussed below.

Computerised Tomography

As an Adjunct to Surgical Staging

There have been several reports on the CT findings in ovarian carcinoma and the role of CT in its diagnosis and management (Schaner et al. 1977; Amendola et al. 1981; Mamtora and Isherwood 1982; Johnson et al. 1983). In a large series of patients Johnson et al. (1983) demonstrated that CT compared favourably with surgical staging in the pelvis and abdomen (Tables 3 and 4) and was superior to clinical examination of the pelvis and abdomen by experienced physicians (Tables 5 and 6). Disease at the predicted sites of metastases could be demonstrated (Figs. 4, 5, 6 and 7). While surgical staging was the most important investigation it did not identify all the sites of disease. Six patients who had had their liver inspected and palpated were shown to have metastases on CT. Uterine involvement, confirmed at repeat laparotomy, and retroperitoneal lymphadenopathy were other sites of disease missed at initial surgery but identified on CT. Blaquiere and Husband (1983) reported patients with liver metastases identified only on CT and Rosenoff et al.

Table 3. Correlation between results of CT and examination of the pelvis at surgery ($n=48$)

Site	Removed prior to CT	CT and surgery −ve	CT and surgery +ve	CT +ve, surgery −ve	CT −ve, surgery +ve
L. ovary	36	7	4	1	0
R. ovary	36	6	6	0	0
Uterus	20	9	17	2	0
L. pelvis	0	30	16	1	1
R. pelvis	0	32	15	0	1

From Johnson et al. (1983) *Radiology* 146: 447-452

Table 4. Correlation between results of CT and examination of the abdomen at surgery ($n=43$)

Site	CT and surgery −ve	CT and surgery +ve	CT +ve, surgery −ve	CT −ve, surgery +ve
Liver tumour	31	3	6	3
Ascites	33	7	3	0
Abdominal mass	32	10	0	1
Tumour in para-aortic lymph nodes	37	1	3	2
Mesenteric disease	38	3	0	2

From Johnson et al. (1983) *Radiology* 146: 447-452

Table 5. Correlation between results of CT and clinical examination of the pelvis ($n=121$)

Site	Removed prior to CT	CT and clinical exam. −ve	CT and clinical exam. +ve	CT +ve, clinical exam. −ve	CT −ve, clinical exam. +ve
L. ovary	80	25	11	2	1
R. ovary	83	21	13	1	1
Uterus	48	21	35	13	2
L. pelvis	0	60	45	15	0
R. pelvis	0	66	43	10	0

From Johnson et al. (1983) *Radiology* 146: 447-452

Table 6. Correlation between results of CT and clinical examination of the abdomen ($n=108$)

Site	CT and clinical exam. −ve	CT and clinical exam. +ve	CT +ve, clinical exam. −ve	CT −ve, clinical exam. +ve
Liver tumour	81	6	18	0
Ascites	69	21	18	0
Abdominal mass	68	31	6	1
Tumour in para-aortic lymph nodes	95	0	11	0
Mesenteric disease	98	2	5	0
Other	63	28	14	0

From Johnson et al. (1983) *Radiology* 146: 447-452

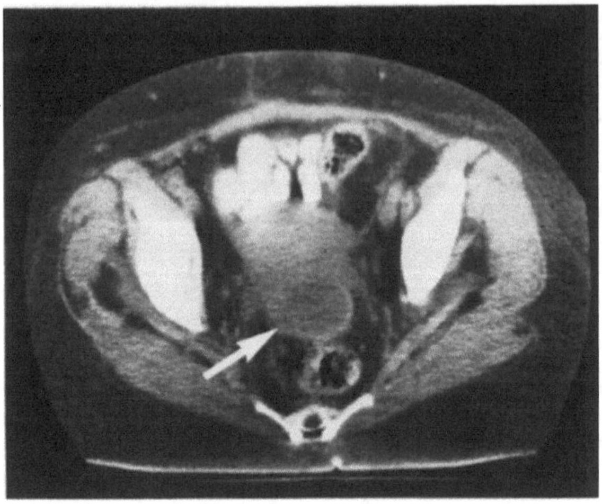

Fig. 4. CT scan demonstrating a cystic metastasis in the pouch of Douglas involving the uterus (arrowed)

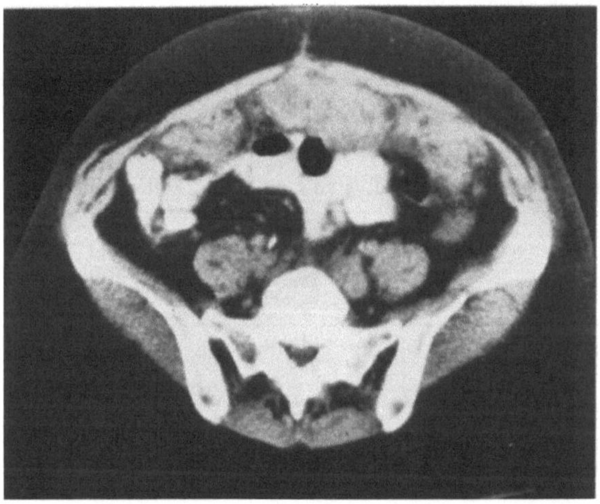

Fig. 5. CT scan demonstrating metastatic disease of the greater omentum. There is a large mixed-density mass extending across the abdomen beneath the anterior abdominal wall

(1975) found diaphragmatic metastases on peritoneoscopy in 7 out of 16 patients thought to have disease localised to the pelvis at laparotomy. The detection of unsuspected disease is important as it may alter the choice and efficacy of subsequent therapy. Additional staging procedures are therefore warranted. CT is a non-invasive procedure comparing well with surgery and capable of imaging all the predicted sites of metastases. As such it is a useful adjunct to surgical staging.

The ability of CT to be used as a single non-invasive staging technique assumes greater importance when those patients who have had inadequate surgical staging and procedures are considered. Only a third of patients referred to a regional oncology centre in the North-West of England had had adequate surgical staging combined with total abdominal hysterectomy, bilateral salpingo-oophorectomy and omentectomy (Table 7). In addi-

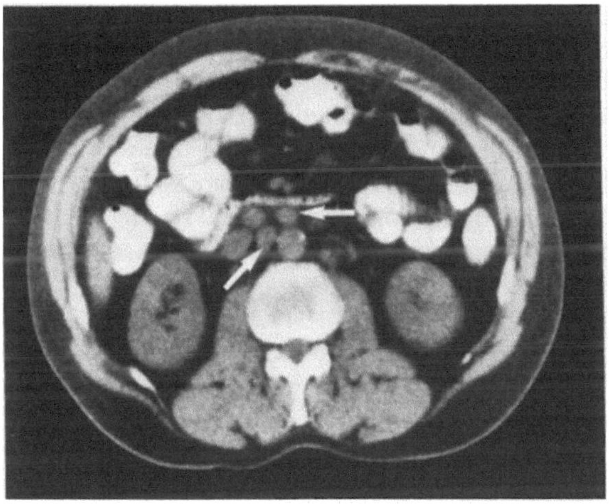

Fig. 6. CT scan demonstrating retroperitoneal lymphadenopathy. There are enlarged para-aortic and para-caval nodes (arrowed)

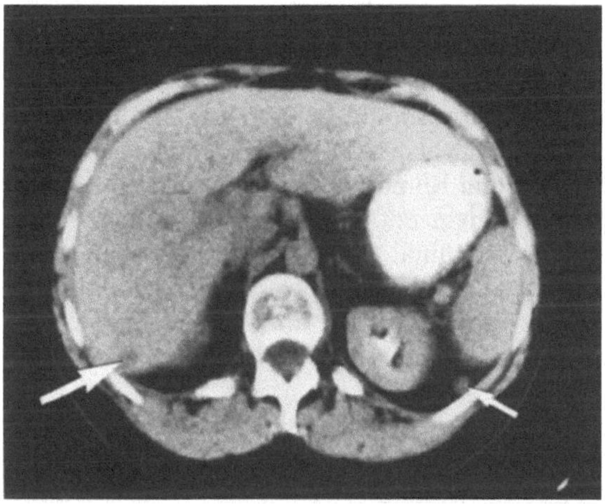

Fig. 7. CT scan demonstrating a focal lesion in the posterior aspect of the right lobe of the liver (large arrow). There is a 1-cm diameter peritoneal deposit under the left hemi-diaphragm (small arrow)

Table 7. Surgical procedures in patients referred to the Manchester Ovarian Cancer Group Trial

Procedure	No.	%
TAH, BSO and omentectomy + debulking[a]	29	32
TAH and BSO + debulking	16	17
BSO + debulking	19	21
Biopsy only	16	17
Other (i.e. debulking only)	12	13
Total	92	100

[a] TAH, total abdominal hysterectomy; BSO, bilateral salpingo-oophorectomy

tion to staging CT will provide objective measurements of disease in order to assess response to additional treatment, or information that enables a repeat laparotomy combined with adequate debulking procedures to be undertaken (Mamtora and Isherwood 1982; Johnson et al. 1983). Several of the patients detailed in Table 7 who were thought to have had adequate surgery with nil or only minimal residual disease were found to have bulk tumour on the CT scan prior to chemotherapy. This may be related to rapid tumour growth after surgery and is a further indication for additional staging.

If radiotherapy is the proposed treatment following surgery then the CT scan may assist in radiotherapy planning (Blaquiere and Husband 1983).

Re staging; Assessment of Tumour Response; Further Surgery

Assessment of the end point of treatment in ovarian carcinoma is difficult. Surgery with adequate debulking improves survival (Griffiths 1975) and post-operative radiation therapy is valuable in the treatment of stage II ovarian carcinoma, improving 5-year survival (Tobias and Griffiths 1976). Recently the introduction of combination chemotherapy combined with surgical procedures has led to the realisation that long-term survival may be possible in advanced disease (Young et al. 1978; Griffiths et al. 1979). The use of complex and aggressive chemotherapy regimes in advanced ovarian carcinoma requires more sophisticated techniques than clinical examination for assessing the response to treatment and detecting the end point of therapy. Peritoneoscopy and second-look laparotomy are methods currently employed. At second-look laparotomy it may be possible to resect residual tumour and determine whether chemotherapy should be stopped or continued (Smith et al. 1976). Removal of remaining gynaecological organs, which are sites for recurrent disease, may also improve survival (Wallach and Blinick 1970).

However, the practice of second-look laparotomy is not universally established. Peritoneoscopy, although useful for assessment of abdominal and pelvic disease when performed by experienced personnel, is an invasive procedure and potentially hazardous in the presence of adhesions following surgery and radiotherapy. It does not permit visualisation of the retroperitoneum and may miss residual tumour deep within the pelvis (Fisher and Young 1977).

CT is able to visualise the retroperitoneum as well as other areas in the abdomen and pelvis and is superior to clinical examination. These factors make it a useful technique for assessing response to therapy, especially in patients with advanced disease (Amendola et al. 1981; Mamtora and Isherwood 1982; Johnson et al. 1983; Blaquiere and Husband 1983). Although the limitations of CT prevent the identification of residual tumour less than 1 cm in diameter a negative CT scan is a guide for clinicians in deciding when to stop therapy, especially if second-look laparotomy is not routinely undertaken. Identification of resudual or progressive disease not detected clinically will lead to modification or continuation of therapy. Whilst a negative CT examination does not preclude second-look laparotomy at institutes where this is routine (Stern et al. 1981; Maggino et al. 1983; Goldhirsch et al. 1983), the CT findings can influence the timing of the second-look procedure and may identify patients in whom further surgery is not warranted e. g. those with residual bulk tumour involving multiple bowel loops.

Previously inoperable disease predicted to be operable on the CT scan or the isolated finding of an abnormal uterus may be an indication for further surgery if this is not otherwise contemplated (Johnson et al. 1983).

Ultrasound

US findings in advanced ovarian carcinoma have been reported (Requard et al. 1981; Paling and Shawker 1981) and there are several comparisons of CT and US as staging techniques (Cosgrove et al. 1980; Coulam et al. 1982; Sanders et al. 1983).

Cosgrove et al. (1980), using laparotomy as the yard-stick, found that CT and US were accurate techniques in the assessment of residual pelvic disease following chemotherapy. In the abdomen, US was unreliable except in the detection of liver metastases. There was a high scan failure rate and peritoneal seedlings and omental deposits were not detected. Coulam et al. (1982) found that CT was more accurate than US in establishing the presence of disease of the pelvic side wall, the involvement of other pelvic organs and the detection of lymphadenopathy. Both CT and US could detect small amounts of ascites. Sanders et al. (1983) found that in general CT was more accurate than US in predicting the tumour stage although the difference was not significant. These studies indicate that CT has certain advantages over US in assessing the extent of disease in the abdomen and pelvis. Whilst providing similar information in the pelvis and liver, CT is better at identifying disease within the peritoneum and in the retroperitoneum.

The limitations of both techniques are similar. Neither will characterise tissue or detect lesions less than 1 cm in diameter, particularly peritoneal seedlings and lymph node metastases. Although the introduction of water-soluble contrast medium into the peritoneum may enhance the detection of peritoneal deposits by CT (Dunnick et al. 1979) it is not likely to overcome the problem. Loops of bowel within the pelvis, adherent to each other or to pelvic organs, may cause interpretive error on US examination and on the CT scan, particularly if in the latter situation they have not been adequately opacified with oral contrast medium. Examination with real-time US equipment may solve the problem as to whether there is a tumour mass present. The post-operative appearance in the region of the vault of the vagina can also cause interpretive errors on both CT and US scanning.

If access to a CT scanner is limited then US will provide a useful staging investigation, especially if assessment of the pelvis and the liver is required. In those centres that rely on CT scanning US may be useful in distinguishing unopacified bowel loops from tumour or other pelvic organs. A further role for US is in guiding needle drainage procedures for loculated ascites.

Lymphography

The lymphatics are a recognised pathway for the spread of ovarian carcinoma. The lymphatics of the ovary follow the ovarian veins and on the right ascend to lymph nodes in the para-caval region at the level of the second and third lumbar vertebrae. On the left the lymphatics drain into nodes in the renal hilar and para-aortic areas at the level of the first lumbar vertebra. Accessory lymphatic channels may drain to the external iliac nodes. Extension of ovarian carcinoma to other pelvic organs provides additional pathways of lymphatic spread. Tumour cells within the peritoneum will flow preferentially to the lymphatics of the right hemi-diaphragm and then to the mediastinal nodes.

Detection of lymph node involvement is important, especially in patients with stage I and II disease, as it may alter the choice of additional therapy. Knapp and Friedman (1974) performed aortic node biopsy in 26 patients with apparent stage I ovarian carcinoma and found a 19% incidence of metastases. They did not think it feasible on the basis of palpation alone to determine whether grossly enlarged nodes contained tumour or whether normal-sized nodes were free of tumour. They therefore recommended routine biopsy of retroperitoneal nodes as part of surgical staging. This is now accepted practice.

Bipedal lymphography is used in many centres to detect lymph node involvement by primary and secondary malignancy. Its accuracy in detecting lymph node involvement in ovarian carcinoma is documented, with an incidence of lymph node metastases ranging from 8% to 22% in stage I; 5% to 20% in stage II; 29% to 41% in stage III; to more than 50% in stage IV disease (Hanks and Bagshaw 1969; Fuchs 1969; Parker et al. 1974; Musumeci et al. 1980). In the series reported by Musumeci et al. (1980), the lymphography findings were compared with histology in 96 patients. Radiological accuracy was confirmed in 33 of 33 positive and 55 of 63 negative lymphograms and of the 8 false-negative examinations, 5 were due to the presence of micrometastases.

The newer imaging modalities of CT and US will detect lymph node metastases. The criterion for tumour involvement on CT and US is the presence of an enlarged node. Metastases in normal-sized nodes will not be detected and if the node is enlarged due to a reactive or inflammatory process, it would be falsely regarded as involved by tumour. Lymphography will estimate node size and internal architecture and is, therefore, capable of detecting metastases in normal-sized nodes. Follow-up radiographs are an important part of the procedure, as initially negative examinations may become positive (Mac Donald 1982). Equivocal lymphograms can be further evaluated by fluoroscopically guided percutaneous needle biopsy (Dunnick et al. 1980). The disadvantages of lymphography compared with CT and US are that it is an invasive procedure, time-consuming and associated with complications, although these are infrequent. Certain lymph node areas which are the sites of metastases will not be imaged by conventional lymphography. These include the internal iliac nodes, nodes at the renal hilum and those in the upper abdomen and retrocrural space.

The use of lymphography varies at different centres. As mentioned above, its role in pre-operative staging is controversial. The majority of patients will undergo surgery, at which time biopsy of pelvic, para-aortic and para-caval nodes should be undertaken. It could be argued that pre-operative identification of abnormal nodes, particularly if of normal size, may guide the surgeon as to which nodes to biopsy. However, lymphography will miss micrometastases, and if it is carried out on all patients suspected of having ovarian carcinoma, an unnecessary and invasive procedure will be performed on a number of patients with a benign condition. As well as the time and cost involved, patients will have been subjected to some discomfort prior to undergoing major surgery. Post-operatively, several centres rely on the non-invasive techniques, particularly CT, as an adjunct to surgical staging or in the assessment of response to treatment. Lymphography would appear to be most valuable in identifying metastases in normal-sized nodes in those patients with stage I and II disease in whom surgery and CT have not identified disease outside the pelvis. In the absence of nodal metastases, these patients may be treated by pelvic radiotherapy or, in certain categories of stage I disease, by follow-up only. There are no reports on the incidence of metastases in normal-sized nodes not identified at surgery or by CT in patients with stage III and IV disease. Such findings are unlikely to affect the immediate management of the patient. Even so, some centres may feel it is justifiable to document the lymph node status by lymphography after additional treatment, especially if second-look laparotomy is not undertaken.

Summary

Surgery is the most important staging technique in ovarian carcinoma. However, in some patients bulk disease may be missed and other patients will have had inadequate staging and surgical procedures. Additional investigations are important in detecting unsuspected disease and providing baseline measurements of residual disease prior to further treatment. Despite its known limitations CT scanning is an accurate non-invasive technique for doing this. Awareness of the post-operative appearances in the pelvis and the use of real-time US scanning when there are unopacified bowel loops will reduce the number of interpretive errors.

Ultrasound is a useful technique for assessing disease in the pelvis and liver and can be used when access to a CT scanner is limited. It is less reliable than CT at detecting disease within the peritoneum and retroperitoneum.

Lymphography is of most value in patients with apparent stage I and II disease in whom surgery and CT scanning have not demonstrated lymph node metastases.

References

Amendola MA, Walsh JW, Amendola BE, Tisnado J, Hall DJ, Goplerud DR (1981) Computed tomography in the evaluation of carcinoma of the ovary. J Computer Assisted Tomography 5 (2): 179-186

Bagley CM Jr, Young RC, Canellos GP, DeVita VT (1972) Treatment of ovarian carcinoma: possibilities for progress. N Engl J Med 287: 856-862

Bagley CM Jr, Young RC, Schein PS et al. (1973) Ovarian carcinoma metastatic to the diaphragm: Frequently undiagnosed at laparotomy. A preliminary report. Am J Obstet Gynecol 116: 397-400

Barber HRK, Graber EA (1971) The postmenopausal palpable ovarian syndrome. Obstet Gynecol 38: 921-923

Bast RC Jr, Klug TL, St John E, Jenison E, Niloff JM, Lazarus H, Berkowitz RS, Leavitt T, Griffiths CT, Parker L, Zurawski VR, Knapp RC (1983) A radioimmunoassay using a monoclonal antibody to monitor the course of epithelial ovarian cancer. N Engl J Med 309: 883-887

Blaquiere RM, Husband JE (1983) Conventional radiology and computed tomography in ovarian cancer: Discussion paper. J R Soc Med 76: 574-579

Bryan PJ, Butler HE, LiPuma JP, Haaga JR, El Yousef SJ, Resnick MI, Cohen AM, Malviya VK, Nelson AD, Clampitt M, Alfidi RJ, Cohen J, Morrison SC (1983) NMR Scanning of the Pelvis: initial experience with a o.3 T system. AJR 141: 1111-1118

Campbell S, Goessens L, Goswamy R, Whitehead M (1982) Real-time ultrasonography for Determination of ovarian morphology and volume. A possible early screening test for ovarian cancer? Lancet I: 425-426

Cancer Facts and Figures (1975) American Cancer Society, New York

Cosgrove DO, Barker GH, Husband JE, McCready VR, Pussell SJ, Wiltshaw E (1980) Carcinoma of the ovary: An evaluation of the role of ultrasound and CT scanning in its management. In: T Wagai, R Omoto, VR McReady (eds) Ultrasound in medicine and biology. Proceedings of the second meeting of the World Federation for Ultrasound in Medicine and Biology. Excerpta Medica International Congress Series 505. Excerpta Medica/Elsevier, New York Amsterdam, pp 25-29

Coulam CM, Julian CG, Fleischer A (1982) Clinical efficacy of CT and US in evaluating gynecologic tumors. Appl Radiol [Jan/Feb]: 79-87

Cutler SJ, Myers MH, Green SB (1975) Trends in survival rates of patients with cancer. N Engl J Med 293: 122-124

Day TG Jr, Smith JP (1975) Diagnosis and staging of ovarian carcinoma. Semin Oncol 2: 217-222
DeLand M, Fried A, van-Nagell JR, Donaldson ES (1979) Ultrasonography in the diagnosis of tumours of the ovary. Surg Gynecol Obstet 148: 346-348
Dunnick NR, Jones RB, Doppman JL, Speyer J, Myers CE (1979) Intraperitoneal contrast unfusion for assessment of intra-peritoneal fluid dynamics. AJR 133: 221-223
Dunnick NR, Fisher RI, Chu EW, Young RC (1980) Percutaneous aspiration of retroperitoneal lymph nodes in ovarian cancer. AJR 135: 109-113
Fisher RI, Young RC (1977) Advances in the staging and treatment of ovarian cancer. Cancer 39: 967-972
Fleisher AC, Everette James A Jr, Millis JB, Julian C (1978) Differential diagnosis of pelvic masses by gray scale sonography. AJR 131: 469-476
Fuchs WA (1969) Malignant tumours of the ovary. In: WA Fuchs, JW Davidson, HW Fischer (eds) Lymphography in cancer. Recent results in cancer research 23. Springer-Verlag, Berlin Heidelberg New York
Goldhirsch A, Triller JK, Greiner R, Dreher E, Davis BW (1983) Computed tomography prior to second look operation in advanced ovarian cancer. Obstet Gynecol 62: 630-634
Griffiths CT (1975) Surgical resection of tumour bulk in the primary treatment of ovarian carcinoma. Natl Cancer Inst Monogr 42: 101-104
Griffiths CT, Parker LM, Fuller AF Jr (1979) Role of cytoreductive surgical treatment in the management of advanced ovarian carcinoma. Cancer Treat Rep 63: 235-240
Hanks GE, Bagshaw MA (1969) Megavoltage radiation therapy and lymphangiography in ovarian cancer. Radiology 93: 649-654
Hricak H, Alpers C, Crooks LE, Sheldon PE (1983) Magnetic resonance imaging of the female pelvis: Initial experience. AJR 141: 1119-1128
Johnson RJ, Blackledge G, Eddleston B, Crowther D (1983) Abdomino-pelvic computed tomography in the management of ovarian carcinoma. Radiology 146: 447-452
Julian CG, Woodruff JD (1969) The role of chemotherapy in the treatment of primary ovarian malignancy. Obstet Gynecol Surv 24: 1307-1342
Kabawat SE, Bast RC Jr, Welch WR, Knapp RC, Colvin RB (1983) Immunopathologic characterization of a monoclonal antibody that recognizes common surface antigens of human ovarian tumours of serous, endometrioid, and clear cell type. Am J Clin Pathol 79: 98-104
Knapp RC, Friedman EA (1974) Aortic lymph node metastases in early ovarian cancer. Am J Obstet Gynecol 119: 1013-1017
Kobayashi M (1976) Use of diagnostic ultrasound in trophoblastic neoplasm and ovarian tumours. Cancer 38: 441-452
Lawson TL, Albarelli JN (1977) Diagnosis of gynecologic pelvic masses by gray scale ultrasonography: Analysis of specificity and accuracy. AJR 128: 1003-1006
Levi S, Delval R (1976) Value of ultrasonic diagnosis of gynecologic tumours in 370 surgical cases. Acta Obstet Gynecol Scand 55: 261-266
Lewis E, Zornoza J, Jing BS, Chuang VP, Wallace S (1982) Radiologic contributions to the diagnosis and management of gynecologic neoplasms. Semin Roentgenol 17 (4): 251-268
MacDonald JS (1982) In: TB Kinmouth (ed) The lymphatics, 2nd edn. Edward Arnold, London, p 351
Maggino T, Ronsisvalle O, Tredese F, Valente S, Brandes A, Onnis GL, Marchesoni D (1983) Role of computed abdominal tomography (CAT scan) in the follow up of ovarian tumours. Eur J Gynaecol Oncol 4 (1): 47-49
Mamtora H, Isherwood I (1982) Computed tomography in ovarian carcinoma: Patterns of disease and limitations. Clin Radiol 33: 165-171
Marglin SI, Castellino RA (1981) Radiologic staging of ovarian carcinoma: Necessary or redundant? Int J Radiat Oncol Biol Phys 7: 1091-1093
McGowan L, Stein DB, Miller W (1966) Cul-de-sac aspiration for diagnostic cytologic study. Am J Obstet Gynecol 96: 413-417
McGowan L (1978) Ovarian cancer. In: L McGowan (ed) Gynecologic oncology. Appleton-Century-Crofts, New York, pp 283-331

Meire HB, Farrant P, Guha T (1978) Distinction of benign from malignant ovarian cysts by ultrasound. Br J Obstet Gynaecol 85: 893-899
Morley P, Barnett E (1970) The use of ultrasound in the diagnosis of pelvic masses. Br J Radiol 43: 602-616
Moyle JW, Rochester D, Sider L, Shrock K, Krause P (1983) Sonography of ovarian tumours: Predictability of tumour type. AJR 141: 985-991
Munnel EW (1968) The changing prognosis and treatment in cancer of the ovary. Am J Obstet Gynecol 100: 790-805
Musumeci R, De Palo G, Kenda R, Tesoro-Tess JD, Di Re F, Petrillo R, Rilke F (1980) Retroperitoneal metastases from ovarian carcinoma: Reassessment of 365 patients studied with lymphography. AJR 134: 449-452
OPCS Mortality Statistics (1982)
Paling MR, Shawker TH (1981) Abdominal ultrasound in advanced ovarian carcinoma. J Clin Ultrasound 9: 435-441
Parker BR, Castellino RA, Fuks ZY, Bagshaw MA (1974) The role of lymphography in patients with ovarian cancer. Cancer 34: 100-105
Requard CK, Mettler FA Jr, Wicks JD (1981) Preoperative sonography of malignant ovarian neoplasms. AJR 137: 79-82
Rosenoff SH, De Vita VT, Hubbard S, Young RC (1975) Peritoneoscopy in the staging and follow up of ovarian cancer. Semin Oncol 2: 223-228
Sanders RC, McNeil BJ, Finberg HJ, Hessel SJ, Siegelman SS, Adams DF, Alderson PO, Abrams HL (1983) A prospective study of computed tomography and ultrasound in the detection and staging of pelvic masses. Radiology 146: 439-442
Schaner EG, Head GL, Kalman MA, Dunnick NR, Doppman JL (1977) Whole body computed tomography in the diagnosis of abdominal and thoracic malignancy: Review of 600 cases. Cancer Treat Rep 61: 1537-1560
Schwartz PE, Weiner M (1979) Ultrasound in gynecology: A clinician's viewpoint. In: Genitourinary ultrasonography clinics in diagnostic ultrasound 2. pp 183-190
Smith JP, Delgado G, Rutledge F (1976) Second look operation in ovarian carcinoma. Cancer 38: 1438-1442
Stern J, Buscema J, Rosenshein N, Siegelman S (1981) Can computed tomography substitute for second look operation in ovarian carcinoma? Gynecol Oncol 11: 82-88
Tobias JS, Griffiths CT (1976) Management of ovarian carcinoma. Current concepts and future prospects (part I of II). N Engl J Med 294: 818-823
Wallach RC, Blinick G (1970) Second look operation for carcinoma of the ovary. Surg Gynecol Obstet 131: 1085-1089
Walsh JW, Taylor KJW, Wasson JFM, Schwartz PE, Rosenfield AT (1979) Grey-scale ultrasound in 204 proven gynecologic masses: accuracy and specific diagnostic criteria. Radiology 130: 391-397
Walsh JW, Rosenfield AT, Jaffe CC, Schwartz PE, Simeone J, Dembner AG, Taylor KJW (1978) Prospective comparison of ultrasound and computed tomography in the evaluation of gynecologic pelvic cases. AJR 131: 955-960
Watring WG, Edinger DD, Anderson B (1979) Screening and diagnosis in ovarian cancer. Clin Obstet Gynaecol 22: 745-757
Young RC, Chabner BA, Hubbard SP, Fisher RI, Bender RA, Anderson T, Simon RM, Canellos GP, DeVita VT Jr (1978) Advanced ovarian adenocarcinoma. A prospective clinical trial of melphalan (L-PAM) versus combination chemotherapy. N Engl J Med 299: 1261-1266

Radioimmunoscintigraphy

K. E. Britton, M. Granowska, and J. H. Shepherd*

Department of Nuclear Medicine and Department of Gynaecology, St. Bartholomew's Hospital, London EC1, United Kingdom

Introduction

Techniques for imaging cancer become more sophisticated yearly. Some, such as ultrasound and computerised tomography, depend on the physical differences between cancer tissue and normal tissue, the tumour size and its effects on surrounding tissue. Others, such as nuclear magnetic resonance, depend on the alteration of the water content of cancer tissue. Radionuclide imaging of cancer has previously relied on alteration of metabolism in surrounding tissues, such as bone, or on non-specific uptake, as with the concentration of gallium-67 citrate.

That cancerous tissue differs from normal body tissue is self-evident. One problem has been to define the nature of this difference and more specifically to demonstrate features of the cancer cell that do not occur in the normal cell. The search for such determinants has led to the identification of some cancer-associated substances, including alphafetoprotein (Goldenberg et al. 1980a), carcinoembryonic antigen (CEA) (Mach et al. 1980) and human chorionic gonadotrophin (HCG) (Begent et al. 1980). In this search, antibodies to such substances have been developed and indeed labelled with radioactive tracers in order to try and image the site of the cancer and its metastases in man. Although there is a long way to go until an ideally specific antibody is produced which is capable of identifying a particular cancer cell, encouraging progress has been made in localising radioactive tracers on malignant tissue for imaging purposes and potentially for therapy.

The Antibody

Three types of approach to the development of antibodies for labelling have been made. They are to develop antibodies against circulating components, against surface components present in cancer cells, or against normal cell components that are hidden or remote from blood. The disadvantage of using circulating components such as CEA and HCG is that, in addition to their low specificity, some part of any injected antibody may be taken up in the blood and prevented from reaching the tumour. The possibility of sensitisation reactions to immune complex formation then arises. The antigen should therefore prefer-

* The support of the Imperial Cancer Research Fund is gratefully acknowledged. The text is based on publications in *Nuclear Medicine Communications, Radiology Nuclear Medicine Images* and *Monoclonal Antibodies for Tumour Detection and Drug Targeting* (Academic Press (London) Ltd)

Ovarian Cancer, Ed. by N. M. Bleehen

ably be fixed to the cell surface as integral part of that surface. However, such cancer-specific antigens are not known and surface antigens that are common to several cancers and/or normal tissues such as placental alkaline phosphatase are used as substitutes. The third approach is to use an antigen that is a constituent of the normal cell but one that is not normally exposed to blood: for example, a component of an epithelial surface lining. Only with the excessive growth and architectural disruption that characterises malignant change would such an epithelial surface antigen be exposed to circulating blood and therefore able to take up sufficient of the labelled antibody.

The epithelial surface lining of the duct of the lactating breast contains an antigen called the human milk fat globule (HMFG), which is found in human milk from which lipid has been removed. This antigen is also present in the epithelial surface of the colon and the lining cells of the ovarian follicles. It is a high-molecular-weight (>300 K) glycoprotein (Burchell et al. 1983) and has been shown to consist of at least 50% carbohydrate (Shimizu and Yamauchi 1982). It seems to be a mucin-like molecule with a high serine, threonine and proline content and O-linked sugars. Against this antigen, a monoclonal antibody HMFG-2 has been developed.

Monoclonal Antibody

The production of antibody has undergone a revolution that has made progress in this field rapid. The conventional method of production is to inject an extract of tissue containing the antigen into an appropriate animal and then repeat this injection at, for example, weekly intervals to boost the immune response. This response consists of the production of stimulated lymphocytes and a whole range of antibodies varying in immunoglobulin class, avidity and specificity. Such a mixture of antibodies is termed 'polyclonal' as it comes from a variety of immune cells.

Kohler and Milstein (1975) demonstrated a technique for isolating and culturing individual immune cells produced in such a response so that each cell becomes the head of a family, or clone, of similar offspring. Normally such a clone would have limited survival. They were able to impart immortality to such immune cells through fusion of the cells with a line of myeloma cells from the same animal, initially the mouse. The 'hybridoma' cells made of the fusion of the myeloma and the immune cells were shown each to produce one particular antibody of one class, called a 'monoclonal' antibody. Then by a process of screening and selection, the clone producing the most suitable monoclonal antibody in terms of avidity or specificity is selected and cultured. The result is a continuous production of a single species of antibody of homogenous quality and definable characteristics in potentially unlimited amounts. The search is on for such monoclonal antibodies with the specificities and avidity required for individual cancer detection. Such antibody would then be suitable vehicles on which to target therapy, either in the form of a particle-emitting radionuclide or a toxin like ricin, to and against the cancer cell (Hazra and Dass 1983).

The hybridoma producing HFMG-2 was derived from the fusion of the mouse myeloma cell line NSI with the spleen cells of a mouse which had received an initial injection of HMFG followed by a boost with cultured normal milk epithelial cells (Taylor-Papadimitriou et al. 1981). By immunoperoxidase staining of formalin-fixed, paraffin-embedded sections the spectrum of reactivity of the antibody has been determined (Arklie et al. 1981). It reacts with primary and metastatic breast tumour, ovarian cancer and colonic cancer and weakly with some normal epithelial cells. The antigenic site recognised by HMFG-2 is present only infrequently on the extracellular mucin-like molecule secreted by the lactating (and other secretory) epithelial cells, but it is more common in the cell membrane of many tumours, particularly those of breast and ovarian origin (Burchell et al. 1983; Taylor-Papadimitriou et al. 1984). The binding of HMFG-2 to HMFG can be inhibited by the lectins peanut agglutinin, wheat germ agglutinin and *Limumus polyhemus,* which are specific for GalB1-3GalNAc, B (1-4)GlcNAc and sialic acid respectively. These results indicate that the antigen may be carbohydrate in nature. The antibody is of the IgG1 class.

The Radionuclide Label

In order to demonstrate the localisation of the antibody in vivo an appropriate radioactive label is required. The choice of label depends on the physical properties of available radionuclides, and their suitability for labelling antibodies (Table 1).

^{131}I (iodine) has the disadvantage that 80% of the radiation emitted is as beta rays. The long half-life means also that only a relatively small amount of activity can be given since the radiation dose is related to the product of the activity given and the half-life. The high energy of the gamma radiation penetrates the thin crystal of the modern gamma camera so the efficiency of count collection is poor. However, the ready availability, cheapness, and ease of labelling with ^{131}I commend it as the label with which new studies are commenced.

^{123}I has an energy ideal for the gamma camera and a short half-life which allows a count rate to be obtained which is about one hundred times that obtained with ^{131}I for the same administered activity. Its availability, however, is limited, usually to once weekly, and in lower activity than ^{131}I. It is also costly. For labelling, added stable iodine carrier is necessary to push the reaction to completion. Thus synthesis of the labelled antibody is a little more difficult than with ^{131}I.

The labelling of antibody with iodine has been a standard procedure for decades, since ^{125}I-labelled antibody is the cornerstone of the in vitro radioimmunoassay procedures for the measurement of hormones and other substances. The chloramine T and Iodogen techniques are the ones most frequently used, the latter being the chemically milder of the two methods. The essential requirement is to label the antibody at a site away from the active centre so as not to affect its immunospecificity. To this end a 1:1 iodine to antibody molar ratio is recommended.

Table 1. Radionuclides for Radioimmunoscintigraphy

Radionuclide	Gamma ray (keV)	Beta rays	Suitability for:		Half-life	Availability
			Gamma camera	Antibody labelling		
^{131}I	364	Present	Poor	Very good	8 days	Any day
^{123}I	159	Absent	Excellent	Good	13 h	Once weekly
^{111}In	171	Absent	Good	Moderate	67 h	Twice weekly
^{99}Tc^{m}	140	Absent	Excellent	Poor	6 h	Twice daily

The use of iodine-labelled antibody has some disadvantages. The patient requires loading with stable iodine (usually in the form of potassium iodide 60 mg twice daily from the day before, and for 3 days after the study for ^{123}I and for 2 weeks after for ^{131}I. The metabolism of iodine-labelled antibody in vivo is relatively rapid and about 20% free iodine is liberated in 24 h. However, it is evident from animal studies that the iodine label attached to antibody bound to tumour does not come off (Epenetos et al. 1982b) and it is the unbound labelled antibody that is metabolised. However it does matter whether the iodine is bound or free in blood or tissues other than the cancer, as it all contributes to the background 'noise' against which the signal from the cancer is to be determined.

^{111}In (Indium) has a suitable energy for detection by the gamma camera but its gamma ray flux is considerably less than that of ^{123}I. Its longer half-life has the potential commercial advantage that there would be time for a manufacturer to label, undertake quality control, package and distribute ready-labelled antibody to centres undertaking radioimmunoscintigraphy. The labelling procedure is more complex and requires the use of bifunctional chelate, one end of which binds the Indium and the other the protein. The cyclic anhydride of diethylenetriamine pentaacetate (DTPA) is a satisfactory chelate for this purpose (Paik et al. 1983). ^{111}In-labelled antibody is less rapidly metabolised in the body (c. 5% per 24 h) than radioiodine-labelled antibody. However, a higher than expected liver uptake of the ^{111}In-labelled antibody may be seen. Free ^{111}In is bound to plasma transferrin and [^{111}In]DTPA is excreted in the urine.

^{99}Tc^{m} (technetium) is the most commonly used radionuclide in nuclear medicine imaging as it can be produced on site from a generator. However, it has two major disadvantages in this context. It is particularly difficult to label biologically active proteins so that they remain stable in vivo for 24 h, and its short half-life of 6 h means that too little activity is present at the time of maximum antibody uptake (which is usually between 12 and 24 h).

The key requirements for the monoclonal antibody are specificity and avidity. The higher the specificity the more antibody will bind to the tumour, always provided that there are sufficient antigenic sites available. Conversely the non-target normal tissue background will be lower. Even more important is the avidity of the antibody, where not only its initial binding strength to the surface antigen but also its staying power for remaining attached to the antigen is crucial. An adequate residence time is essential if delayed imaging is to be undertaken.

There are two imaging strategies for radioimmunoscintigraphy. The first is to image early at a time of maximum uptake of the labelled antibody, that is up to 24 h, using a short-half-life high-count-rate radionuclide label in order to give maximum sensitivity. However, the higher normal tissue activity may require correction using a background subtraction or target enhancement technique. This may be done by injecting a blood pool agent and subtracting its distribution from that of the labelled antibody (Goldenberg et al. 1980b). There are major theoretical and practical problems due to the difference between the gamma ray energy of the blood background agent (e.g. ^{99}Tc^{m}) and that of the antibody label (e.g. ^{131}I) (Green et al. 1984). A variation of this technique is to subtract an early static image taken at around 10 min from later images at for example, 4 and 24 h after injection of the isotope. This requires accurate patient and image repositioning techniques and the use of change detection algorithms to recognise and test for significant differences between the early, mainly blood pool image and the late image which contains the sites of uptake of the labelled antibody. This approach is showing promise (Granowska et al. 1983). The alternative is to use single photon emission tomography (SPET) to separate target tumour from other tissues.

The second strategy is to image late using a longer-lived radionuclide such as ^{131}I. Since labelled antibody fixed to the tumour keeps up its signal strength while the other tissue and blood background activity is falling away due to metabolism and loss with time, the target to non-target ratio improves with time after peak uptake. However, the total count rate is relatively low with ^{131}I and falls further with time so that statistical noise may obscure the image. The staying power of the antibody on the tumour's antigenic sites is also time dependent. As a result the first strategy using ^{123}I or ^{111}In and early scan time is gaining favour.

Labelling with ^{123}I

^{123}I has a half-life of 13 h, produces no beta rays and its gamma rays have an energy of 159 keV, which is ideal for the gamma camera. The iodogen reaction is used with ^{123}I to label the monoclonal antibody. Iodogen is dissolved in dichloromethane to make iodogen solution and evaporated to dryness at 37 °C in sterile propylene tubes. Iodogen reagent is then left coating the inside of the tube, which can be stored at 5 °C for 6 months without loss of reactivity. The following technique is then used for labelling antibody (Granowska et al. 1984). Pure ^{123}I, the HMFG-2 antibody and potassium iodide are mixed in the iodogen tube. Potassium iodide is added because it is necessary to increase the ionic strength of the iodine for the labelling reaction to proceed to completion.

The pH is adjusted to 8.5 using sodium borate and the mixture left at room temperature for 10 min with gentle shaking. The mixture is then decanted onto a Sephadex G50 filtration column in a 20-ml syringe prewashed with 1% human serum albumin in phosphate-buffered saline. After a 5-ml void volume, the eluate is collected in 2-ml aliquots, activity assayed and passed through a micropore filter into sterile vials.

Quality control is undertaken using 10-μl samples from before and after gel filtration. They are spotted at the origin of 10-cm absorbent strips which are then developed in an ascending manner with 10% trichloroacetic acid. The radioactivity of the strips is determined. The labelling efficiency is typically over 80%. Iodinated protein is precipitated at origin and free ^{123}I is at the solvent front. Reactivity of iodinated antibody with tumour cell extract is tested using an enzyme-linked immunosorbent assay (ELISA). It is shown that this iodogen method leaves the active centre of the antibody intact with its avidity unaltered (Epenetos et al. 1982a).

Patient Protocol

Patients were under the care of a gynaecologist (J. S.), having been referred with suspected or known ovarian cancer. They were aged between 30 and 75 years old. The procedure was explained and each gave signed consent. Potassium iodide (60 mg twice daily) was given orally the day before and for 3 days after the study. A skin test with the antibody was performed before the study to test for allergy. The patients were divided into four groups:

Group 1 Patients with a mass in the abdomen or pelvis of undiagnosed cause but for which there was a reasonable clinical suspicion that it could be due to ovarian cancer.

Group 2 Patients with clinically obvious ovarian cancer in whom the aim was to determine the extent of the disease before operation. The extent of the disease was determined at surgery in order to 'stage' the ovarian cancer.

Group 3 Patients who had been operated on for ovarian cancer elsewhere, having histological proof of the disease, but who had been referred for specialist treatment at our gynaecology/oncology unit. The extent of the disease as determined by antibody imaging was compared with that determined by other techniques such as ultrasound and computerised tomography.

Group 4 Patients with ovarian cancer who had already undergone complete or incomplete surgical resection of disease and had received chemotherapy. In some of these a second-look operation was necessary to determine the extent of any residual disease as a guide to further treatment. In others chemotherapy had failed and re-operation was indicated.

The patient lies supine on the scanning couch and a gamma camera is placed over the pelvis anteriorly. The injection of 2–3 mCi of ^{123}I-labelled monoclonal antibody containing 0.5 mg of antibody is given intravenously. Dynamic studies are recorded for the first 10 min directly into the computer. Static images are then taken, anteriorly and posteriorly of the whole of the abdomen, together with marker scans. These are also transferred directly into the computer. The procedures are repeated at 4 h and 22 h. The patient then proceeds to surgery later that morning.

One of the problems with this type of imaging is that the detail of tumour may not be clear and then a technique of background correction is required. The method empolyed in this study is to subtract the 10-min image from the 4-h and the 22-h images, using radioactive markers placed on the patient to coordinate the two pictures. Transparent films of the marker positions on the persistence scope are made at the early visit, and the patient's skin marked. At each subsequent visit the markers are relocated on the patient and the patient is positioned until the image of the marker on the persistence scope coincides with that on the previously recorded film placed over the scope. The computer is also programmed so that the recorded images can be moved and fixed one pixel at a time, vertically, horizontally or by rotation, so that an exact superimposition of the later image over the earlier image may be made. Although many primary ovarian tumours and their metastases may be seen without background subtraction, the use of this subtraction technique has resulted in the unequivocal identification of metastases with relatively low uptake (Granowska et al. 1983).

Results

The results are given for the first 40 patients studied. Two of the early patients who were only imaged for the first 4 h were incorrectly diagnosed. Two patients with colon cancer also showed positive results, because the antibody is not absolutely specific for ovarian cancer, but reacts with colon and breast cancer as well (Epenetos et al. 1982 a). Two patients with tumours thought histologically to be benign (a mucinous cystadenoma and a teratoma) who showed high uptake of the labelled monoclonal antibody, were classified as poor results for group 1. The results are summarised in Table 2 where they are compared with the surgeon's assessment at operation and follow-up. They are illustrated by the following case histories.

A 52-year-old woman presented with a mass in the pelvis (group 1, clinical stage IV). High uptake focally was seen in the centre of the pelvis (Fig. 1). At operation a right ovarian and central pelvic mass was found to involve the colon. Histology showed a poorly differentiated adenocarcinoma.

Table 2. Radioimmunoscintigraphy of ovarian cancer

Independent assessment	Clinical grouping				
	1	2	3	4	Total
Poor	2	–	–	1	3
Equivocal	1	–	–	1	2
Good	4	13	6	12	35
					40

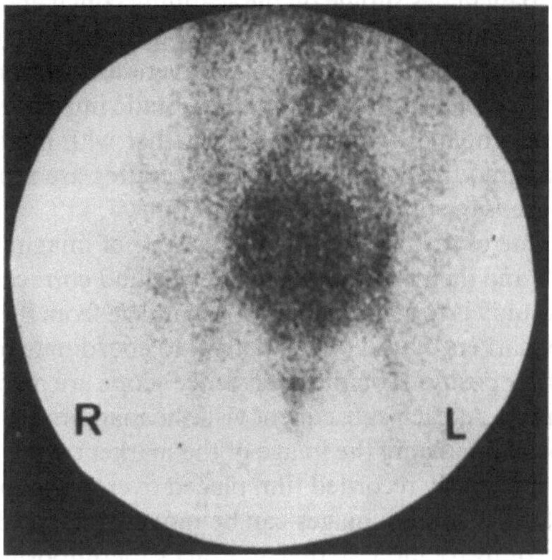

Fig. 1. Radioimmunoscintigraphy image of anterior pelvis at 22 hours shows massive uptake in an ovarian cystadenocarinoma. (By courtesy of *Radiology Nuclear Medicine Images*, published by Nickerson and Collins, Illinois)

A 52-year-old patient presented with pleural effusions and abdominal swelling (group 2, clinical stage IV). Radioimmunoscintigraphy showed uptake in the chest (Fig. 2a). The area above the diaphragm, seen in the posterior view 10-min image, was filled with activity in the 21-h image. Central abdominal and pelvic uptake was evident on the posterior view 21-h image as compared with the 10-min image (Fig. 2b). The surgical exploration confirmed these findings.

A 65-year-old patient presented with pleural effusions and abdominal swelling (group 3, clinical stage III), and at laparotomy there were generalised peritoneal deposits. Subsequent radioimmunoscintigraphy showed widespread uptake. The 10-min image (Fig. 3) showed a 'halo' of ascitic fluid. By 24 h this had increased activity in it, as well as uptake in the pelvis and the region of the omentum. At surgery omental metastases, ascites and diffuse pelvic involvement were seen.

A 64-year-old woman presented with a mass in the left iliac fossa having previously had a total hysterectomy, bilateral salpingo-oophorectomy and partial colectomy for adenosquamous carcinoma of the ovary (group 4, clinical stage IV). Radioimmunoscintigraphy showed uptake in the mass in the left iliac fossa with a central defect and abdominal

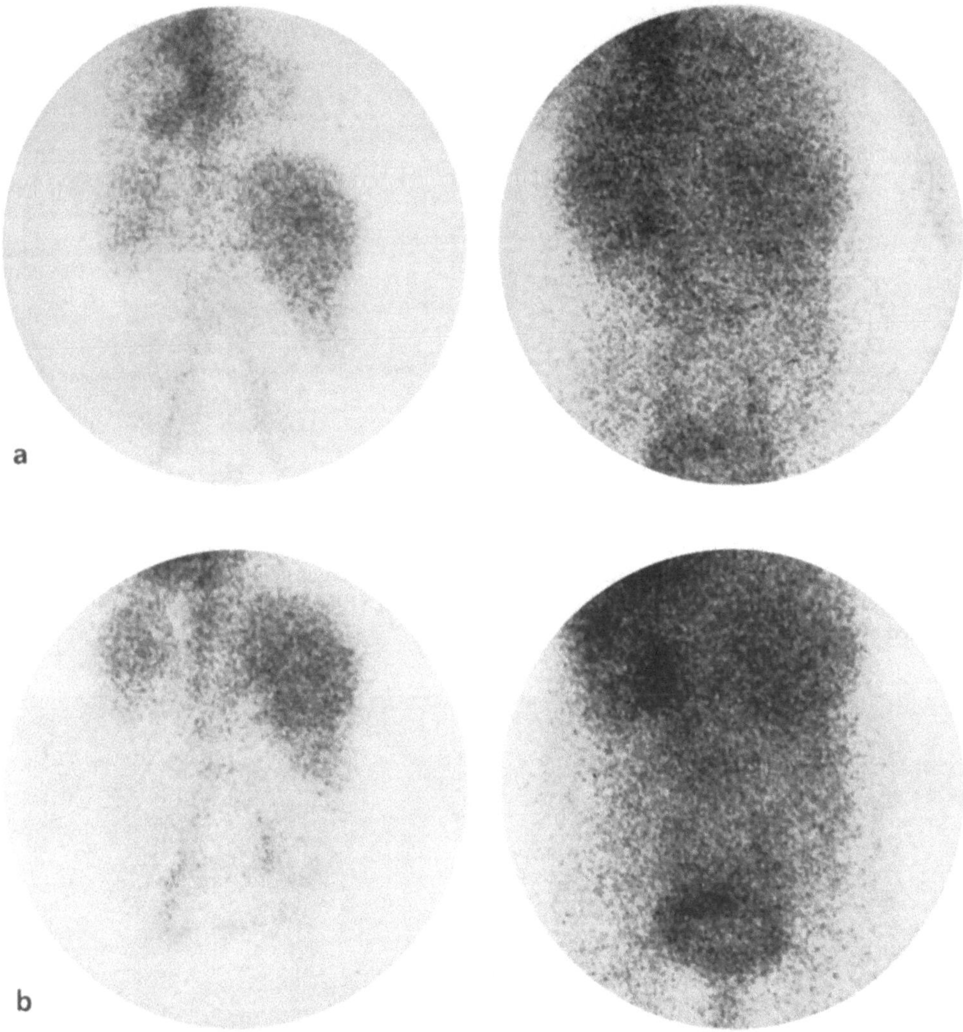

Fig. 2 a, b. **a** Posterior radioimmunoscintigraphy images (left, 10 min; right, 22 h) of lower chest and abdomen. Uptake in the lower chest in malignant pleural effusions and in the mid abdomen is seen on the later image as compared with the early one. **b** Posterior pelvic views (left, 10 min; right, 21 h). Uptake in the central pelvic mass is evident on the late image. (From Granowska et al. (1984) *Nucl Med Comm* 5: 485–499, published by Chapman and Hall, London)

central uptake (Fig. 4). At operation the left pelvic mass was found to be due to lymph node enlargement with central tumour necrosis; para-aortic node involvement was also found.

Discussion

The correlation of imaging results with surgical findings in the 40 patients was good (35/40, 87.5%), and even better if the two patients imaged only for 4 h are excluded. These results confirm those reported by Epenetos et al. (1982 a). Two benign tumours, a muci-

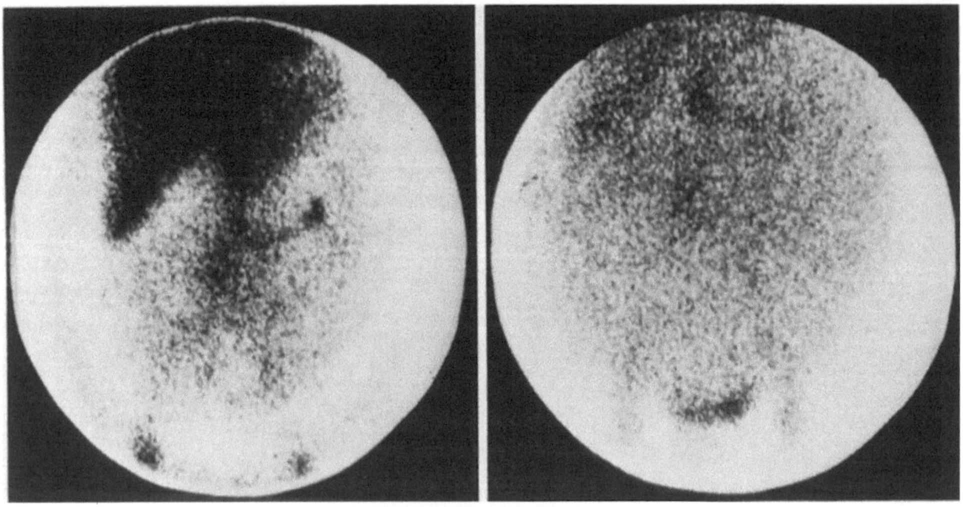

Fig. 3. Radioimmunoscintigraphy images of anterior abdomen (left, 10 min; right, 24 h). The sharp liver outline and inferior 'halo' effect are due to ascites. At 24 h there is general uptake in the malignant ascites due to peritoneal deposits. (From Granowska et al. (1984) *Nucl Med Comm* 5: 485-499, published by Chapman and Hall, London)

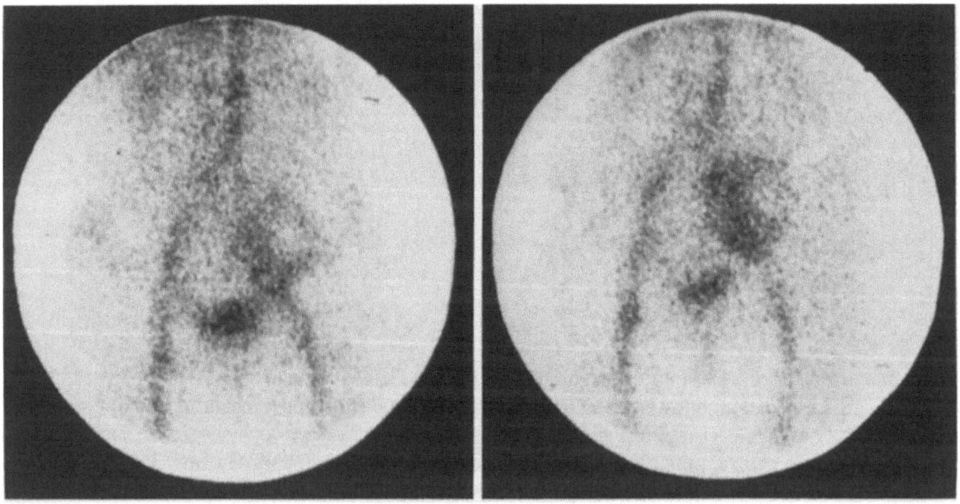

Fig. 4. Radioimmunoscintigraphy images of the anterior abdomen (left, 4 h; right, 24 h). Uptake is shown in the mass on the left; the lateral defect is due to tumour with a necrotic centre. (From Granowska et al. (1984) *Nucl Med Comm* 5: 485-499, published by Chapman and Hall, London)

nous cystadenoma and a benign teratoma, showed good uptake and are classified as poor results in the independent assessment (Table 2).

The radioimmunoscintigraphy images (Fig. 1-4) are all direct films taken from the gamma camera without any processing, background subtraction or other manipulation. They illustrate the effectiveness of the high count rates obtained using ^{123}I, in spite of total tumour uptake being a small fraction of the injected activity (for example 2.4% in one patient). The visual comparison of the later images with the 10-min image usually identifies the sites of specific uptake. The problems of patient repositioning, early background subtraction to enhance the later images, and superimposition of the early on later images have been overcome in a simple way (Carroll et al. 1984). This approach overcomes the difficulties inherent in using a second radioisotope of a different energy as a tissue background or blood pool marker (Goldenberg et al. 1980b; Mach et al. 1981) and it is expected that it can be refined still further using sophisticated programming techniques (Nimmon et al. 1984).

Present monoclonal antibodies are against antigens that are tumour-associated rather than tumour-specific and usually only 2%–3% of the injected dose is taken up by the tumour, with a maximum of 7% to date. It is therefore clear that the advances in this field will come from the development of antibodies of much greater tumour specificity and avidity rather than better radionuclide labels. What matters most is the binding to and staying power on the cancer antigen of the radiopharmaceutical. It is becoming evident that there are two options for imaging: the first is to use a high-count-rate, short-half-life compound to catch the peak of uptake of the antibody by the tumour at around 12–24 h with high sensitivity, but at the cost of a higher blood and tissue background; or to wait until the target to background ratio is maximal, for example at 5 days, at the expense of low count rates, low sensitivity and thus higher statistical noise when using a longer-lived label such as ^{131}I. With background subtraction using both early and late images with accurate computer-assisted repositioning techniques or single photon emission tomography, enhanced early images may be obtained.

In conclusion, the use of ^{123}I-labelled monoclonal antibody is generally successful in ovarian cancer in imaging the primary tumour and metastases in the abdomen, but less successful in determining whether a pelvic tumour is benign or malignant. Its clinical application may be mainly in avoiding the need for a second-look operation to determine the presence or absence of residual metastases after chemotherapy. Tumour-specific rather than tumour-associated antibodies will be required if therapy with alpha- or beta-emitting radiolabelled antibodies or immunotoxins is to be considered in the future.

References

Arklie J, Taylor-Papadimitriou J, Bodmer W, Egan M, Millis R (1981) Differentiation antigens expressed by epithelial cells in the lactating breast are also detectable in breast cancers. Int J Cancer 28: 23–29

Begent RHI, Stanway G, Jones BE, Bagshawe KD, Searle F, Jewkes RF, Vernon P (1980) Radioimmunolocalisation of tumours by external scintigraphy after administration of ^{131}I antibody to human gonadotrophin: Preliminary communications. J R Soc Med 73: 624–630

Burchell J, Durbin H, Taylor-Papadimitriou J (1983) Complexity of expression of antigenic determination, recognized by monoclonal antibodies HMFG-1 and HMFG-2, in normal and malignant human mammary epithelial cells. J Immunol 131: 508–513

Carroll MJ, Flatman WD, Nimmon CC, Granowska M, Britton KE (1984) Congruent image registration as a prerequisite for detecting sequential changes during radioimmunoscintigraphy. Nucl Med Comm 5: 230–231

Epenetos AA, Britton KE, Mather S, Shepherd J, Granowska M, Taylor-Papadimitriou J, Nimmon CC, Durbin H, Hawkins LA, Malpas JS, Bodmer WF (1982a) Targeting of iodine-123-labelled tumour-associated monoclonal antibodies to ovarian, breast and gastrointestinal tumours. Lancet II: 999–1005

Epenetos AA, Nimmon CC, Arklie J, Elliott AT, Hawkins LA, Knowles RW, Britton KE, Bodmer WF (1982b) Radioimmunodiagnosis of human cancer in an animal model using labelled tumour associated monoclonal antibodies. Br J Cancer 46: 1-8

Goldenberg DM, Kim EE, Deland F, Spremulli E, Nelson MO, Gockerman JP, Primus FJ, Corgan RL, Alpert E (1980a) Clinical studies on the radioimmunodetection of tumors containing alpha-fetoprotein. Cancer 45: 2500-2505

Goldenberg DM, Kim EE, Deland FH, Bennett S, Primus FJ (1980b) Radioimmunodetection of cancer with radioactive antibodies to carcino-embryonic antigen. Cancer Res 40: 2984-2992

Granowska M, Shepherd J, Britton KE, Ward B, Mather S, Taylor-Papadimitriou J, Epenetos AA, Carroll MJ, Nimmon CC, Hawkins LA, Bodmer WF (1983) Ovarian cancer diagnosis using I-123 monoclonal antibody in comparison with surgical findings. J Nucl Med 24: P15

Granowska M, Shepherd J, Britton KE, Ward B, Mather S, Taylor-Papadimitriou J, Epenetos AA, Carroll MJ, Nimmon CC, Hawkins LA, Flatman WD, Horne T, Bodmer WF (1984) Ovarian cancer: Diagnosis using 123-I monoclonal antibody in comparison with surgical findings. Nucl Med Comm 5: 485-499

Green AJ, Begent RHJ, Keep PA, Bagshawe KD (1984) Analysis of radio-immunodetection of tumours by the subtraction technique. J Nucl Med 25: 96-100

Hazra DK, Dass S (1983) Choice of radionuclide for antibody labelling: new prospectives. Nucl Med Comm 4: 40-53

Kohler G, Milstein C (1975) Continuous cultures of fused cells secreting antibody of pre-defined specificity. Nature 256: 495-497

Mach J-P, Carrel S, Forni M (1980) Tumour localisation of radiolabelled antibodies against carcinoembryonic antigen in patients with carcinoma. N Engl J Med 303: 5-10

Mach J-P, Buchegger F, Forni M, Ritschard J, Berche C, Lumbroso J-D, Schreyer M, Girandet C, Accolla RS, Carrel S (1981) Use of radiolabelled monoclonal anti-CEA antibodies for the detection of human carcinomas by external photoscanning and tomoscintigraphy. Immunol Today 2: 239-249

Nimmon CC, Carroll MJ, Flatman WD, Marsden P, Granowska M, Horne T, Britton KE (1984) Spatial probability mapping of temporal change: application to gamma camera quality control and immunoscintigraphy. Nucl Med Comm 5: 231

Paik CH, Ebbert MA, Murphy PR, Lassman CR, Reba RC, Eckelmann WC, Pak KY, Powe J, Steplewski Z (1983) Factors influencing DTPA conjugation with antibodies by cyclic DPTA anhydride. J Nucl Med 24: 1158-1163

Shimizu M, Yamauchi K (1982) Isolation and characterization of mucin-like glycoprotein in human milk fat globule membrane. J Biochem 91: 515-524

Taylor-Papadimitriou J, Peterson JA, Arklie J, Burchell J, Ceriani RC, Bodmer WF (1981) Monoclonal antibodies to epithelium-specific components of the human milk fat globule membrane: Production and reaction with cells in culture. Int J Cancer 28: 17-21

Taylor-Papadimitriou J, Burchell J, Change SE (1984) Use of antibodies to membrane antigens in the study of differentiation and malignancy in the human breast. In: Monoclonal antibodies and cancer. Armand Hammer Symposium, Academic Press, New York London (in press)

Radiation Therapy

R. S. Bush*

The Ontario Cancer Institute incorporating, The Princess Margaret Hospital, Toronto M4X 1K9, Canada

The major objective of this discussion is to present the current survival advantages from using radiation therapy in the management of patients with epithelial cancer of the ovary. To do this will require my including the comparative achievements of surgery and chemotherapy. A second objective is to illustrate how clinical trials can improve our knowledge of a disease. This comes from the detailed data collection which is possible within such studies; the resulting data base allows the formulation of hypotheses and the consequent development of sequential trials to test those hypotheses.

There are a series of questions which I will try to answer. First, what role does radiation therapy have that currently cannot be replaced by any other modality? I will provide evidence that for approximately one-third of patients it is the one adjuvant and adjunctive method which, following surgery, has been shown to improve long-term survival consistent with cure. Second, how important are other modalities in ensuring that the maximum benefit and minimum toxicity are achieved from the use of radiation therapy? Information from the literature relating to surgery will be presented as well as from some current studies investigating the combination of radiation and chemotherapy. Nevertheless, firm data to answer this question are not available. Third, are there any physical or biological mechanisms which can explain success or failure in the survival advantage demonstrated for radiation therapy? The answer is yes. The several components which contribute to this answer will comprise a major part of the discussion. The subjects range from concepts of tumour growth, prognostic groupings of patients (based on post-operative residual bulk, tumour type, grade and stage), the end-points used to measure the effectiveness of any treatment, and the technique of giving radiation therapy.

Ovarian cancer is a complex disease and all of our current treatment methods are potentially toxic. So, to achieve for each patient the maximum gain from treatment, it becomes essential that the various therapeutic modalities are used optimally. I trust that answering the questions posed above will provide a better understanding of what has been achieved by all modalities. Nevertheless, it must be realised that the optimal use of radiation therapy currently yields less than a 10% improvement in long-term survival for all patients with ovarian cancer. The greatest challenge comes from the large proportion of patients who present with extensive bulky disease and for whom cure is unlikely using currently available treatment. Prevention and earlier diagnosis may be the only solutions to this problem.

---

* The author gratefully acknowledges the contribution of his associates at The Princess Margaret Hospital to the results reported in this paper, and in particular the multifactorial analysis of prognostic factors by Dr Dembo. I am also indebted to Miss Attlewhyte for the dedication she has shown in preparing this manuscript

Ovarian Cancer, Ed. by N. M. Bleehen

The discussion will be organised as follows: First, the data relating to the probability of cure will be examined, together with the significance of the necessary criteria. It is important to realise that cure is possible, and that it is dependent upon management decisions. Second, I will examine the reported results of surgery alone, in order to provide a base from which to estimate the effectiveness of adjuvant or adjunctive therapy. Third, the results of various clinical studies will be presented to examine current achievements with radiation therapy, and, where possible, compare them with those using chemotherapy. Fourth, the many prognostic factors which have been recognised will be presented, together with a discussion of their significance, their potential impact on management and the evaluation of outcome.

Probability of Cure

There are two main outcome measurements which can be used to examine the effect of treatment on mortality. These are:

1. *Incidence-mortality data.* These can be used particularly to see whether there is a difference between the reported incidence and mortality. If there is not, it will be very difficult to argue that any patients have been cured.
2. *Survival data.* These are essential, particularly those regarding long-term survival. When patients can be shown to be dying at the same rate as those of the same age in the general population, there is a reasonable expectation that a fraction of the patient population has been cured. This conclusion is strengthened if it can be shown that death from the primary cancer decreases to the same rate as in the general population, or that relapse decreases to zero with time.

I will discuss the information available on these end-points in order to demonstrate the proportion of cured ovarian cancer patients. Other end-points are of little or no value in determining cure (Bush and Dembo 1980; Bush 1984).

Incidence and Mortality

The diagnosis and classification of malignancies affecting the ovary has only been established with any degree of uniformity for the last 15 years. No new pathological types have been proposed since 1968 (Santesson and Kottmeier 1968). Nevertheless the ovary is a common site for metastatic cancer, particularly from stomach, bowel, breast, lung and endometrium. Scully (1970) reported that of those cases presenting as a primary ovarian cancer, approximately 10% will be metastatic. Consequently, there is still some uncertainty about the accuracy of current registry information.

Registry data for some malignancies do show a mortality decrease as might be expected from the response to new treatments, particularly chemotherapy. Data are available, and an example has been reported (Bush 1984) of management changes influencing the relative separation of incidence and mortality. In particular, the mortalities of patients with Hodgkin's disease and testicular carcinoma can be shown to have dropped significantly since the introduction of potentially curative chemotherapy (Clarke 1983: data from Ontario Tumour Registry).

For many years there have been reports of responses of ovarian cancer to chemotherapy, together with arguments for the curative potential of that modality. Such reports have

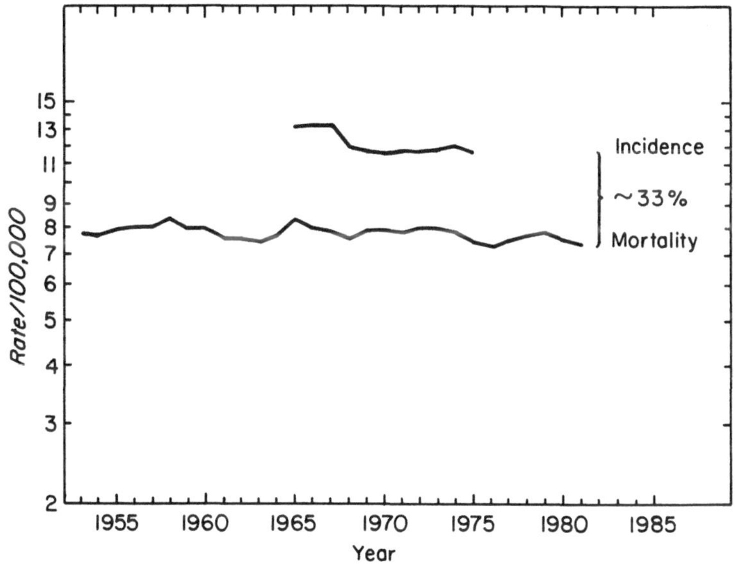

Fig. 1. Ontario incidence and mortality rates for patients classified as having cancer of the ovary. Three-year moving averages; age standardised for world population. Reliable incidence data are available currently only for a 10-year period, 1965–1975. See text for discussion. (With kind permission of the Editor of *Radiology*)

increased in recent years with the introduction of combination chemotherapy, particularly those combinations that include cisplatin. Nevertheless, Ontario mortality data for patients with ovarian cancer show no significant change between the years 1975 and 1981 (Clarke 1983), and this is similar to the data reported by other registries (American Cancer Society 1983). From the separation of incidence and mortality rates in Fig. 1, and assuming there has been no change in the incidence rates since 1975, approximately one-third of patients with cancer of the ovary appear to have been cured in that they do not die of their primary disease. One question which needs to be answered is whether treatment is contributing to this incidence-mortality difference and, if so, which of the modalities, either singly or in combination, it is that is important. This question will be considered later in the discussion. First, a more fundamental question will be answered: that is, whether the separation of incidence and mortality rates indicates that patients are cured. To answer this question survival data need to be examined.

Survival Data

Using the data reported by the International Federation of Gynaecology and Obstetrics (FIGO), an average 5-year survival fo 30% can be calculated for 4812 patients with epithelial cancer of the ovary seen at a variety of centres around the world (Kottmeier 1979). Although the 5-year survival rate is only an estimate of the cure rate, it currently provides a reasonable estimate of the long-term survival, as will be shown below.

The pattern of survival over the 20 years following diagnosis of epithelial cancer of the ovary is shown for Princess Margaret Hospital (PMH) patients in Fig. 2. A large fraction of the 2343 patients die relatively quickly, and at 5 years only 33% are alive. There is then a

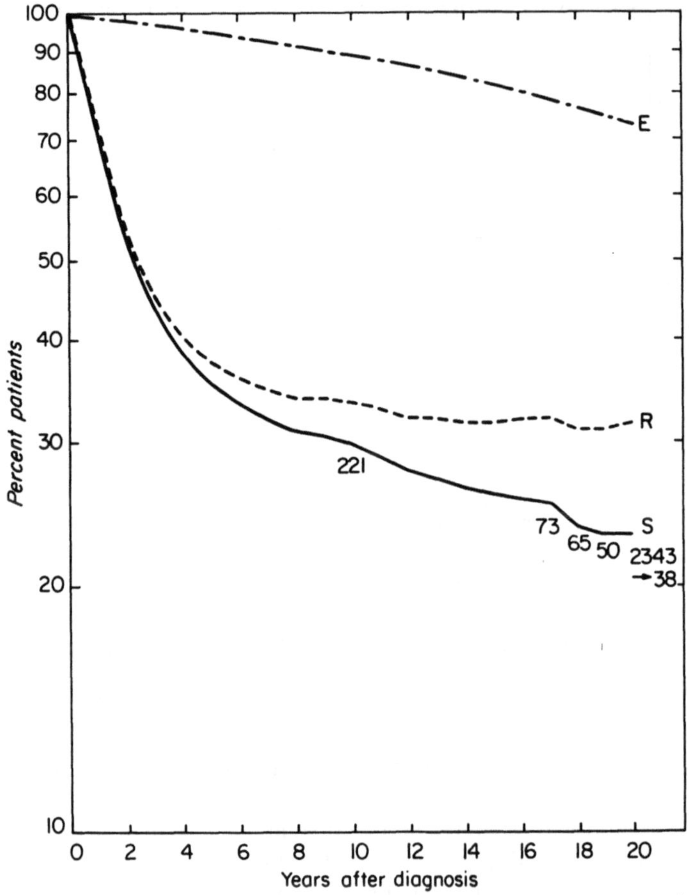

Fig. 2. The actuarial survival (S) of the 2343 patients with epithelial cancer of the ovary seen at the PMH between the years 1958 and 1982 inclusive. Age-adjusted expected survival (E) and relative survival curves (R) are also shown

much slower rate of dying out to 20 years, when 24% are shown to be still surviving. The change in the survival rate with time may be due to changes in the rate of dying from the primary cancer, or from other causes of death, particularly if there is a wide range of age groups in the patient population.

An estimate of the probability of dying from other causes can be obtained by examining the expected survival of the patients if they had not developed cancer. The survival of women in the general population with the same age distribution as the patients is the reference curve. Although the survival of the general population will include the risk of dying from each of the gynaecological malignancies, this risk is small compared with the total of all causes of death (Registrar General of Ontario 1978). There is in this comparison, however, a potential error which occurs with increasing time after diagnosis. This error arises if the probability of controlling the cancer is dependent upon the age of the patient. This is true for patients with cancer of the ovary. Consequently, the age distribution of the surviving treated population will change differently from the way it normally would. To examine the expected survival for the patient population at any point in time, it is necessary to change the age distribution of the reference population at regular intervals to match the age distribution of the surviving patient population (Bush et al. 1982). The age-adjusted expected survival curve (E) in Fig. 2 more accurately reflects the effect on survival at any point in time of causes of death other than cancer of the ovary than does the expected survival curve for the initial age distribution of the patient population.

Survival is plotted on a logarithmic scale in Fig. 2, so that if the actuarial survival curve (S) for patients becomes parallel to the expected (E), the rate of change of each is equal. It can be seen that this appears to be so after approximately 12 years. Confirmation is obtained by calculating a relative survival curve (R). If the relative survival curve becomes parallel to the abscissa, then it confirms that the chance of a patient dying is the same as that of the comparable proportion of the general population, and can be taken as evidence of cure. As shown in Fig. 2 the relative survival curve indicates approximately 31% have been cured. Note that the 5-year survival gives an acceptable, though optimistic estimate (33%) of the final cure rate. The criteria for cure used above would have more weight if supported by evidence that the patients are still not dying from ovarian cancer. Unfortunately, it is only since April 1971 that we have had sufficiently detailed information to establish precisely the causes of death in all patients. The survival curve using death from disease as the end-point (cause-specific survival curve) can be established from that date, and has been shown to be no different from the relative survival curve (Bush et al. 1982).

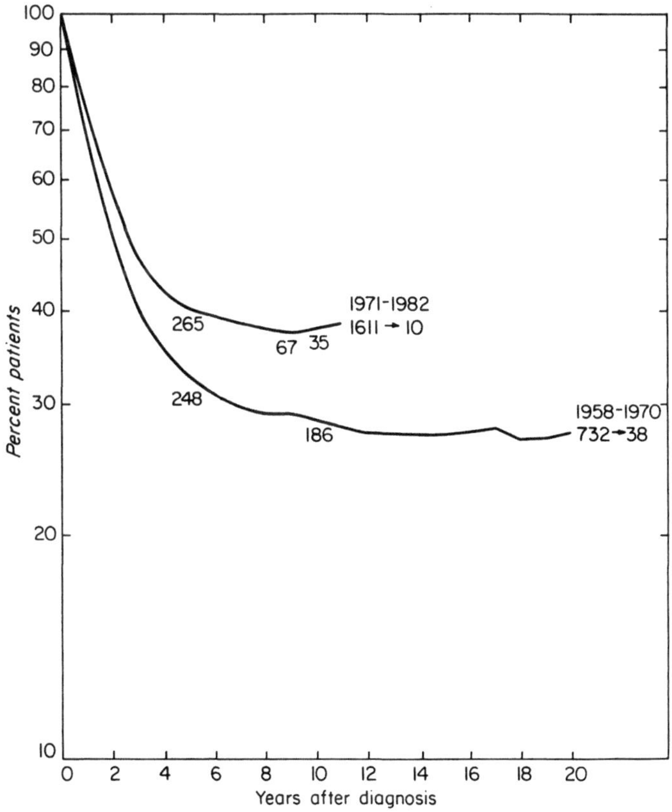

Fig. 3. The relative survival curves for patients with epithelial cancer of the ovary seen at the PMH in two periods of time

Consequently the relative survival curves can be used to determine the cure rate for patients with cancer of the ovary.

Fig. 3 shows the relative survival curves for patients seen between the years 1958 and 1970 inclusive, and also between 1971 and 1982. The relative survival curve for the earlier period indicates a cure rate of 27%-28%. For the later period, although there is apparent flattening at 37%-38%, it is most probably still too early to determine at what level the plateau will finally be established. From the shape of the curve it is to be expected that it will be around 35%-36%. Nevertheless, there is a clear separation of the two curves, indicating an 8%-10% improvement in the long-term survival of patients between the two periods. We have no evidence that the patient population has changed significantly as regards stage, tumour type or grade (Bush and Dembo 1984), and on the basis of our prospective clinical trial results believe that this increase is due to the improved efficacy of our treatment methods. For patients entered into the prospective studies between April 1971 and December 1982 the 5-year survival is 40.3% and for those eligible but not entered it is 40.6%. Patients not eligible for the studies as a result of being referred for consultation only, no laparotomy, active concurrent cancer or previous malignancy have only a 20% 5-year survival. All these groups have been included in the relative survival curve of Fig. 3.

Summary

Evidence has been presented from incidence and mortality data indicating that approximately one-third of patients diagnosed as having cancer of the ovary do not die as a result of this malignancy, and that this has changed little over the last 20-30 years. Survival data on patients in the province of Ontario indicate that the proportion surviving in the long term consistent with their being cured has remained approximately the same, although definitive evidence that it was treatment which influenced survival has not yet been presented. The 5-year survival gives an optimistic estimate of the expected cure rate. The results of the PMH experience suggest that there has been an improvement in survival of patients in that centre with time; this is believed to be due to improved management methods.

Clinical Achievements

For those patients with cancer of the ovary who are rendered disease free at operation, a proportion must be expected to have been cured by surgery. If these patients could be recognised, no adjuvant treatment would be required. The problem in decision-making is that when those patients cannot be clearly identified, an estimate of the proportion which might have been cured has to be made in order to evaluate the effectiveness of adjuvant therapy and decide on the indications for its use. Also, if there is any toxicity from that treatment, it becomes important to determine whether the potential benefit for those with unrecognised residual disease is greater than the price which may have to be paid by those who do not require any further therapy. The following discussion will present evidence that post-operative therapy does contribute to the long-term survival, and also an estimate of the survival from surgery alone.

The analysis of the survival of 808 patients seen, reviewed and eligible for prospective studies between 1971 and 1978 demonstrates a 5-year survival of 38%. Three hundred and eleven (311) patients were classified as having no known residual disease after their initial surgery. This is 38% of the patient population and is the same as the survival estimate. The question which arises from this comparison, is whether all the cures been achieved by the initial surgery. If so, adjuvant or adjunctive radiation and/or chemotherapy would be achieving nothing in curative terms. Let me try to answer that question before going on to try to estimate the cure rate from surgery alone. In the 808 patients mentioned, there were 141 who were known to have residual disease but who were classified as being potentially curable with adjunctive therapy. These patients were clearly not cured by their surgery, and yet following adjunctive therapy the actuarial 5-year survival is 39.5%, and the relapse-free rate 31%. Consequently the cure rate is likely to lie somewhere between these two estimates. The median period of follow-up is 7.43 years, with all patients being followed for 5 years or more. Clearly then, adjunctive therapy has resulted in a proportion of patients that are most probably cured. As this subpopulation of patients with known residual disease is 17.5% of the total population of 808 patients, it can be estimated (using the total population as the denominator) that adjunctive therapy for these patients has provided a 5-year survival of 7%. Thus, surgery alone cannot have provided a 5-year survival greater than 31%, and it is likely to be less than this. This is because, having demonstrated that a proportion of patients with known residuum survive 5 years, it is probable that those patients falsely classified as having no known residuum will also receive a survival benefit from adjuvant therapy. I will now provide an estimate of the survival following surgery alone.

Surgery Alone

Estimates of the 5-year survival rate following surgery can be made, but obviously not verified if there is evidence or belief that further therapy can provide a survival benefit. On the basis of PMH data for patients with stage IA and IB disease and treated by surgery alone, or with inadequate adjuvant therapy, a lower limit of 12% can be established. Using published survival data for surgery alone in all stages of cancer of the ovary (Bagley et al. 1972) with the stage distributions reported by FIGO or those at the PMH, upper limits of 22% and 18% respectively can be set. This estimate then for the surgical cure rate is significantly lower than the fraction of patients rendered clinically disease free by surgery. Somewhere between 12% and 22% are estimated as surviving 5 years, and most probably 20%, or 1 patient in 5, would be a reasonable estimate (Bush and Dembo 1984). The conclusion must be that surgical cures are from those with zero residuum and that adjuvant and adjunctive therapy is raising the overall survival rate to 30%–40%.

The next question to be asked is to what extent, apart from curing a significant fraction of patients, is surgery important in improving the efficacy of the adjuvant and adjunctive therapy? Smith has reported the survival of patients receiving various adjuvant therapies in relation to the amount of postsurgical residual disease (Smith 1980). There is an inverse relationship between size of tumour residuum and survival. The implication is that the objective of the initial surgery must be to debulk the tumour when possible to masses less than 1-2 cm in diameter. This appears to have been confirmed by Griffiths, who has provided evidence that surgical debulking is an appropriately aggressive philosophy of management as long as residual tumour masses are 1.5 cm or less in diameter. Twenty per cent of these patients showed long-term survival with post-operative therapy (Griffiths et al. 1970). Patients in whom masses were 1.6 cm or greater after resection showed a steady rate of dying with time.

Patients who had received their initial surgery elsewhere, but following referral had further surgery in which optimal resection was possible, have a similar survival, that is, approximately 20% in the long term. Thus, it is suggested from these data that optimal debulking allows patients to be moved into a more favourable prognostic category. What is not clear is the proportion of unresectable cases that may be successfully debulked when the appropriate surgical skills are available.

Post-operative Therapy

For many years the only modality in addition to surgery capable of providing symptomatic relief for ovarian cancer patients, a clinical response to treatment, or increased survival, was radiation therapy. Evaluation of the effectiveness of radiation from the older literature is difficult because radiotherapy techniques were variable in the critical parameters of field size, dose to normal and to tumour tissue, and fractionation. Randomised studies were not performed, nor was there any attempt to take into account prognostic factors which might influence outcome. Also end-points for evaluating treatment were not standardised. The introduction of chemotherapy brought another modality capable of providing response, symptomatic relief and possibly an improvement in survival. Nevertheless, similar problems have interfered with the accurate assessment of its value. This section will present the results of selected clinical studies and try to put into perspective the proven achievements of radiation and chemotherapy using long-term survival as the end-point for evaluation. First, however, it is necessary to present information on the spread of ovarian cancer to explain both the success and failure of various management approaches.

One of the advances of the past 10–15 years has been the recognition of the risk of spread of ovarian cancer through the abdominal cavity, and particularly to the diaphragm. Proteinaceous and cellular material in the peritoneal cavity is drained predominantly through the lymphatics of the diaphragm (Feldman and Knapp 1974). The constant movement of the diaphragm is believed to increase the probability of any fluid or cells being pulled towards the diaphragmatic surface. The diaphragm as well as the rest of the abdominal cavity must be examined thoroughly at the time of surgery in order to stage patients accurately. Extent of disease is one important prognostic attribute for deciding on treatment. A significant proportion of patients classified as having localised disease at their initial diagnostic procedure have been reported by several investigators to have unrecognised macroscopic metastases in the upper abdomen when further direct examination was carried out (Bagley et al. 1973).

Improved staging procedures can lead to an apparent improvement in survival by stage which may be interpreted as the result of treatment unless overall survival is examined (Bush and Dembo 1980). This is a very important consideration for patients with cancer of the ovary. The outcome of treatment for a given stage using new techniques of classification is sometimes incorrectly compared with outcome of the same stage using older classification methods. This invariably results in an inflated estimate of the therapeutic benefit of the more recently tested therapy. Secondly, studies which are confined to one or two stages rather than covering all stages fail to address the question of whether the observed improvement in treatment has a real impact on the overall survival of patients (Bush 1979a; Bush and Dembo 1980). Until the advent of chemotherapy, the generally held view of practising gynaecologists was that radiation therapy improved the survival of patients who had extension of disease into the pelvic tissues beyond the ovaries (stage II). There was little evidence for any survival benefit in other stages of the disease. Radiation therapy techniques frequently used only pelvic irradiation. We have confirmed that such treatment, although not optimal, can provide a long-term survival advantage for patients with clinical stage II disease. One of the treatment arms in a prospective study at the PMH included pelvic irradiation to a dose of 4500 cGy in 20 daily fractions over 26–28 days utilising the photon beam from a 22 MeV Betatron and parallel opposed 15 cm^2 fields for patients classified as stage II but with known post-operative residual disease. Such patients would not be expected to have been cured by surgery alone. Nevertheless, of 31 such patients treated with pelvic irradiation with or without additional chlorambucil, 12 have no evidence of relapse having been at risk for 7 years or longer. Chlorambucil was shown in the randomised study to provide no long-term survival benefit. Consequently, for these patients pelvic irradiation clearly appears to have been curative. Nevertheless, as will be shown later, pelvic irradiation is not optimal treatment for such patients, and for patients in stage I when there is no known residuum following surgery, it appears to provide no survival benefit. The evidence for this latter conclusion is given below.

Patients with Stage I Cancer of the Ovary

We have reported the results of a prospective study of the management of patients classified as having stage I A cancer of the ovary (Dembo and Bush 1983). The conclusion was that no post-operative treatment was indicated for those whose malignancy was well differentiated, because survival following surgery alone was close to 100%. Approximately 30% of patients with moderately or poorly differentiated cancers did relapse. Nevertheless, pelvic irradiation did not provide any survival advantage because when pelvic relapse was prevented by such treatment, relapse occurred in the upper abdomen. Consequently if treatment is indicated, the objective must be to control unrecognised disease in both the pelvis and upper abdomen.

The Gynecological Oncology Group (GOG) has studied adjuvant therapy for patients classified as having stage I disease (Hreshchyshyn et al. 1980). As in the PMH study, it was demonstrated that most relapses were distributed throughout the peritoneal cavity. The question which the GOG attempted to answer was whether melphalan or pelvic irradiation reduced the frequency of relapse compared with surgery alone. Unfortunately 49% (82/168) of the patients were removed from the study after randomisation, resulting in major dissimilarities in the distribution of patients in each treatment arm. Consequently, no conclusions can be drawn from the therapeutic comparisons because of the potential bias introduced by this high frequency of withdrawals (Dembo et al. 1981). Nevertheless, as there was no significant difference between either experimental arm and the control, adjuvant therapy conferred no survival benefit over surgery alone.

Neither of these two studies demonstrated any survival benefit for Stage I patients from the post-operative treatments studied. To my knowledge there is no randomised study which has demonstrated any benefit. At the PMH we now follow a policy of recommending treatment to Stage I patients only when the malignancy is poorly differentiated, recognising that the relapse rate without post-operative adjuvant treatment is estimated to be 30%. Consequently the treatment used must be potentially curative for the 30% at risk with no significant toxicity for the 70% who will be treated unnecessarily. On the basis of the information obtained from the prospective studies described below we recommend abdomino-pelvic irradiation. We have no data yet to demonstrate that there is an overall benefit for such patients. Chemotherapy has not been shown to provide any survival benefit and there is a significant risk of leukaemia induction, with the population of patients already cured by surgery being at the greater risk. The use of intraperitoneal radioisotopes clearly appears an attractive strategy for these patients, and their use has been discussed in the literature (Rosenshein et al. 1979). Nevertheless, there is no randomised study to demonstrate the relative benefit for this group of patients.

Studies in Patients with a High Risk of Relapse, but Potentially Curable

Delclos and his associates (Delclos and Quinlan 1969) at the M.D. Anderson Hospital (MDAH) in Houston, Texas, contributed significantly to the development of radiation techniques designed to try to control abdominal spread of ovarian cancer as well as that remaining in the pelvis. These investigators modified the technique used at the Christie Hospital in Manchester of moving strip irradiation to treat the upper abdomen. They confirmed that fewer abdominal relapses occurred compared with those after pelvic irradiation alone. During the same period Smith and co-workers at the MDAH produced evidence that chemotherapy in the form of oral or IV melphalan could produce responses for patients with ovarian cancer which appeared to be associated with long-term survival in a proportion of cases (Smith and Rutledge 1970). This led to a direct comparison of the radiotherapy technique of Delclos with oral melphalan for selected patients with zero or minimal post-operative residuum.

The MDAH Randomised Trial between Post-operative

Irradiation and Chemotherapy. Patients at the MDAH were entered in a randomised trial between post-operative irradiation and chemotherapy between April 1969 and November 1975. The only detailed report was an interim analysis of the 149 patients entered up to May 1974 (Smith et al. 1975). The question being asked was whether chemotherapy or radiation therapy provided the greater benefit for patients who were considered at risk of relapse after surgery but who had no obvious residuum or residual tumour masses greater than 2 cm. A further requirement was that any visible residual disease should not be in areas of the abdomen which might be shielded from irradiation. The radiation technique used a standard source to skin distance, with an upward moving strip starting from below the obdurator foramina and extending to the upper abdomen. Whether the diaphragms were included is still unclear. The dose prescribed was a mid-plane dose of 2600–2800 cGy in 8 fractions with liver and kidney shielding, followed or preceded by pelvic irradiation of 200 cGy in 10 fractions. The chemotherapy arm was oral melphalan 0.2 mg/kg/per day for 5 days every 4 weeks, blood counts permitting. A total of 12 cycles was planned.

Seventy patients were randomised to receive irradiation and 79 chemotherapy. The 5-year survival rates were similar (71% vs 72%), and there was no significant difference by stage. Nevertheless, the toxicity and monetary cost of the irradiation treatment were significantly greater than for those receiving melphalan. Consequently, melphalan was considered the more advantageous treatment method.

The PMH Study for Patients with Stages IB, II and III Asymptomatic Presentations. This initial PMH study started in 1971 has been reported (Bush et al. 1977; Dembo et al. 1979a). For patients with Stage IB and II disease, pelvic irradiation (PEL) according to previous accepted practice (4500 cGy in 20 fractions) was used as a control arm. Two study arms with the aim of preventing relapse in the upper abdomen were investigated. One utilised additional irradiation of the upper abdomen (P+AB) to a dose of 2250 cGy in 10 fractions using a strip technique with no shielding except for limiting the kidney

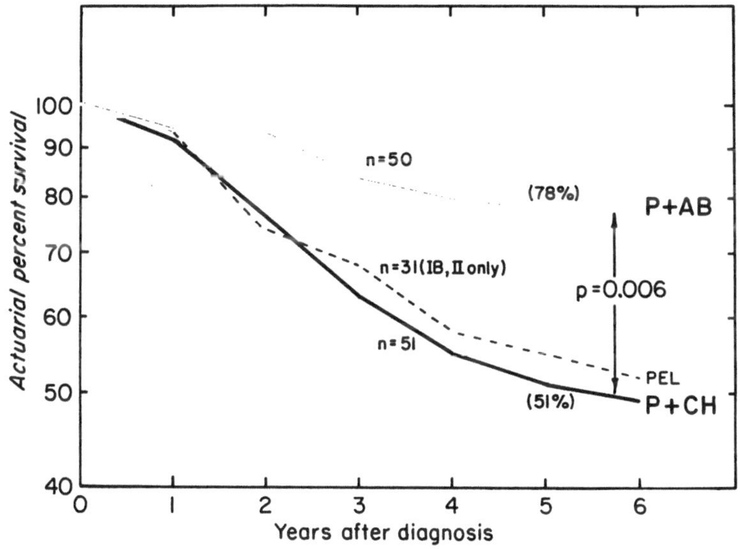

Fig. 4. The results of a prospective randomised trial comparing pelvic and abdomino-pelvic strip irradiation (P+AB) with pelvic irradiation followed by oral chlorambucil for 2 years (P+CH) or pelvic irradiation alone (PEL)

dose to 2000 cGy (Dembo et al. 1979 b). Pelvic irradiation of 2250 cGy in 10 fractions was also presented. The other investigational arm incorporated chlorambucil 6 mg a day for 2 years and pelvic irradiation of 4500 cGy in 20 fractions (P+CH). Stage III asymptomatic patients were randomised only between the two investigational arms, while Stage IB and II patients might also receive the control treatment of pelvic irradiation alone. Fig. 4 illustrates the survival for each treatment arm for those who had had a completed bilateral salpingo-oophorectomy (BSOH comp.). As can be seen the survival was significantly better for P+AB. All treatment groups were comparable with respect to known prognostic factors. Major long-term toxicity with P+AB was uncommon (<5%). Consequently, in this study abdomino-pelvic irradiation with a pelvic boost demonstrated a highly significant survival advantage, compatible with an increase in cure rate, compared with more limited radiation with or without the addition of an alkylating agent.

The abdomino-pelvic irradiation technique used in the PMH study was carefully planned to include the whole peritoneal surface. To achieve this objective required careful consideration of the anatomical landmarks, and appropriate check films were used to ensure that the whole abdomen was irradiated (Dembo et al. 1979 b; Bush 1979 b).

The conclusion from the PMH study has been slow in gaining acceptance. This may be in part due to an inherent resistance to accepting positive study results (Ciampi and Till 1980), but also the result of the MDAH trial may have had a significant influence. It is important, therefore, to examine and compare the details of these two trials to see whether there is any acceptable explanation other than chance for the difference in the conclusions.

The randomised groups in the MDAH study were stratified by pathological type. There was no other stratification built into the study design. This resulted in significantly more stage I or IIA patients in the chemotherapy arm. No information has been provided on comparability between the treatment arms by tumour grade, or the presence or absence of macroscopic tumour residuum. Both these prognostic factors are very powerful, and the lower grades of tumour, and absence of residuum occur more frequently in stages I and IIA than in IIB and III. These observations raise the concern that such powerful prognostic factors may have been unequally distributed and biased in favour of the chemotherapy arm. Consequently the reported survival similarities between the two experimental treatment arms may not be ascribed necessarily to treatment alone (Dembo and Bush 1983).

Important differences also exist between the radiation techniques used at the MDAH and the PMH (Delclos and Quinlan 1969; Bush 1979b; Dembo et al. 1979b). There is considerable doubt that the diaphragm was included in the irradiation field of the MDAH series, and this doubt exists in many reports of the use of whole-abdominal irradiation (Bush 1979b). The inclusion of the diaphragm in the radiation fields used at the PMH, together with the absence of need for liver shielding because of the lower radiation dose, provides a possible explanation to support the positive result for radiation therapy demonstrated in the PMH study.

There was a high complication rate in the irradiation arm of the MDAH study, but this was not so at the PMH. This difference is most probably attributable to the higher radiation dose used at the MDAH, and the greater frequency of more extensive surgical procedures than in Toronto (Delclos and Dembo 1980). A fixed source- to skin distance was used in Houston with patients treated alternately in prone and supine positions. The PMH technique used only the prone position and isocentric fields. We believe and have published evidence that the latter technique provides a more homogeneous dose distribution than that used at the MDAH. This also may have contributed to the lower morbidity rate at the PMH.

This discussion needs also to consider specific major criticisms of the PMH study. There have been two. First, because meticulous surgical staging was infrequently performed, some uncertainty exists as to the equivalence of the true stage distribution between the three treatment arms. Nevertheless, randomisation was used to prevent bias, there were more than 70 patients in each of the two arms which included all three clinical stages, and known prognostic factors were balanced. Only 12 patients were withdrawn after randomisation out of 190 patients entered. Also with a highly significant p value of 0.005, we believe that the probability that the positive result was due to factors other than the treatment variable is highly unlikely. A second criticism is that the results obtained with the abdomino-pelvic radiation arm appeared excellent because of inadequate chemotherapy in one of the other treatment arms. Nevertheless, the survival rates reported for the patients treated with pelvic irradiation and chlorambucil are not lower than those reported for similar patients treated with chemotherapy alone (Bush 1979b; Dembo and Bush 1983).

The most convincing evidence to support the PMH study comes from the PMH trial which was based on those earlier data and conclusions. We compared an open field radiation technique to the PMH strip technique, the latter being the control arm. We have demonstrated that for patients with similar prognostic attributes, survival following the use of the strip technique is the same as demonstrated in the period 1971-76 (Dembo et al. 1983). This preliminary analysis also indicates tumour control is similar and acute toxicity less for the open field technique. The next study underway has the open field technique as the new standard, and examines the value of an increased radiation dose. As will be discussed later, this investigation of a higher dose of radiation is being restricted to those patients identified as having a greater than 70% chance of being cured by the lower dose of radiation. Such a patient subgroup can be recognised now as a result of the extensive data base obtained from this series of sequential studies. Another subgroup previously treated with radiation has a high risk of relapse. For patients so classified, we are investigating the use of combined chemotherapy and radiation in a manner similar to the attempts now being investigated for patients who have gross residual disease after initial surgery. Before discussing the factors used to select patients with different prognose, I will give a brief account of how radiation is being investigated for patients with a low chance of being cured.

Management of Patients with Gross Residual Disease, and a Low Chance for Cure

The 45% of patients who have been recognised as having a poor prognosis are a heterogeneous group. They are characterised by being stage IV, or stages II and III with large residual masses following surgery. They have been treated by a variety of methods. Treatment appears until recently to have achieved only palliation of symptoms with no extension of life. To my knowledge, no study of combination chemotherapy has shown any greater potential for cure than single-agent therapy for this poor prognosis group. Nevertheless, there is now evidence that the median survival of poor prognosis patients may have been increased with the introduction of cisplatin (Sturgeon et al. 1981; Bell et al. 1982; Bush 1984).

Much of the pessimism and frustration which exists in the treatment of patients with ovarian cancer comes from trying to meet the challenge presented by patients in this poor prognosis category. As Lewis and Blessing (1977) observed, 'For ovarian cancer seemingly everything works, but practically nothing succeeds.' In trying to achieve success, attempts are being made by a number of investigators, including those at the PMH, to test combinations of chemotherapy, surgery and radiation. This step has been taken because with chemotherapeutic combinations containing cisplatin the clinical response rate has been significantly higher than with single agents or other combinations. Also an appreciable proportion who have undergone second-look surgery after such chemotherapy have been found to have no detectable disease, microscopic residuum only, or residual masses which have become resectable. It is still not clear whether any significant proportion of these patients has been provided any long-term survival benefit even though there has been such an improvement in response. Because of the lack of long-term success from surgery and chemotherapy in even those patients who demonstrate an excellent response, a number of centres and investigators are examining the value of combining abdomino-pelvic irradiation with post-operative chemotherapy and further surgery when appropriate.

Schwartz and Smith (1980) reported that they had investigated the use of abdomino-pelvic irradiation for patients with small residual disease after melphalan and second-look surgery. Severe myelosuppression occurred when trying to complete the planned radiation therapy. The survival outcome was inferior to that with continued chemotherapy. Melphalan appears to compromise the bone marrow to a greater degree than the combination of cyclophosphamide, adriamycin and cisplatin (CAP). Following six or more courses of this chemotherapeutic regime, we have found it possible to complete whole-abdominal irradiation to greater than 2000 cGy as well as giving a pelvic boost when this is clinically indicated. Similarly Fuks et al. (1982) have reported that aggressive sequential surgery, combination chemotherapy, second-look laparotomy and whole-abdominal radiotherapy are feasible without unacceptable toxicity if carefully planned. Nevertheless, Hainsworth et al. (1983) found that abdomino-pelvic irradiation following intensive combination chemotherapy with cyclophosphamide, adriamycin, hexamethylmelamine and cisplatin produced unacceptable myelosuppression. This was particularly true for patients who experienced significant myelosuppression during the previous chemotherapy. They also noted that there appeared to be little benefit from the radiation therapy for any patient who had clinically evident tumour persisting after initial chemotherapy. They do not recommend radiotherapy under these circumstances. These results are contrary to those reported by Haas et al. (1980).

It is therefore not clear whether abdomino-pelvic irradiation has a significant role to play for any patients with gross residual disease after surgery, but who have had an initial good response to chemotherapy. As Fuks has argued, this is an important question to answer. At the PMH we are investigating this question in a prospective randomised study. We are comparing combination chemotherapy with abdomino-pelvic irradiation for those patients with nil or microscopic residual disease after initial chemotherapy and further debulking if necessary at second-look surgery. We hope also, from this study to establish a much better data base which may allow appropriate selection of patients for any form of aggressive therapy.

Prognostic Factors and Groups

The appropriate categorisation of patients who might benefit from current approaches to management is critical for wise decision-making. Any such categorisation needs to use a multifactorial approach to the combining of prognostic factors to form prognostic groups. Such an approach will be discussed in this final section.

The accurate assessment of the outcome of the treatment of patients with cancer of the ovary is complicated by the effect of multiple prognostic factors. The following are the major ones recognised as having survival significance when examined individually:

1. Stage of disease
2. Pathological type
3. Tumour grade
4. Patient age
5. Residual bulk of disease after surgery
6. Adjunctive/adjuvant therapy

The criteria for staging and pathology classification have changed repeatedly over the years. This causes uncertainty as to whether it is legitimate to compare subgroups of patients from different periods of time. Nevertheless, the FIGO staging has now been unchanged since 1974. The World Health Organisation provides the criteria for the different pathological groups within an accepted classification.

The actuarial survival rates of the 808 patients entered into prospective clinical trials at the PMH between April 1971 and September 1978 are shown in Fig. 5 for the prognostic factors listed above. In the post-operative residuum classification there was an appreciable number of patients for whom it was uncertain whether all identifiable disease had been removed or not. This category is shown as '?' in the figure and is grouped with those classified as having no (0) evidence of residuum. 'Small' residuum refers to clinically evident residual disease, but bilateral salpingo-oophorectomy had been completed. Accurate information on the size of residual masses was not available, but the small residuum rarely exceeded 2 cm in diameter. In the 'large' residuum group the residual masses were invariably larger than 2 cm. Patients were placed in this group if residual disease was present when a complete bilateral salpingo-oophorectomy and hysterectomy had not been performed. This was usually because the bulk or infiltrative nature of the disease prevented the procedure being completed.

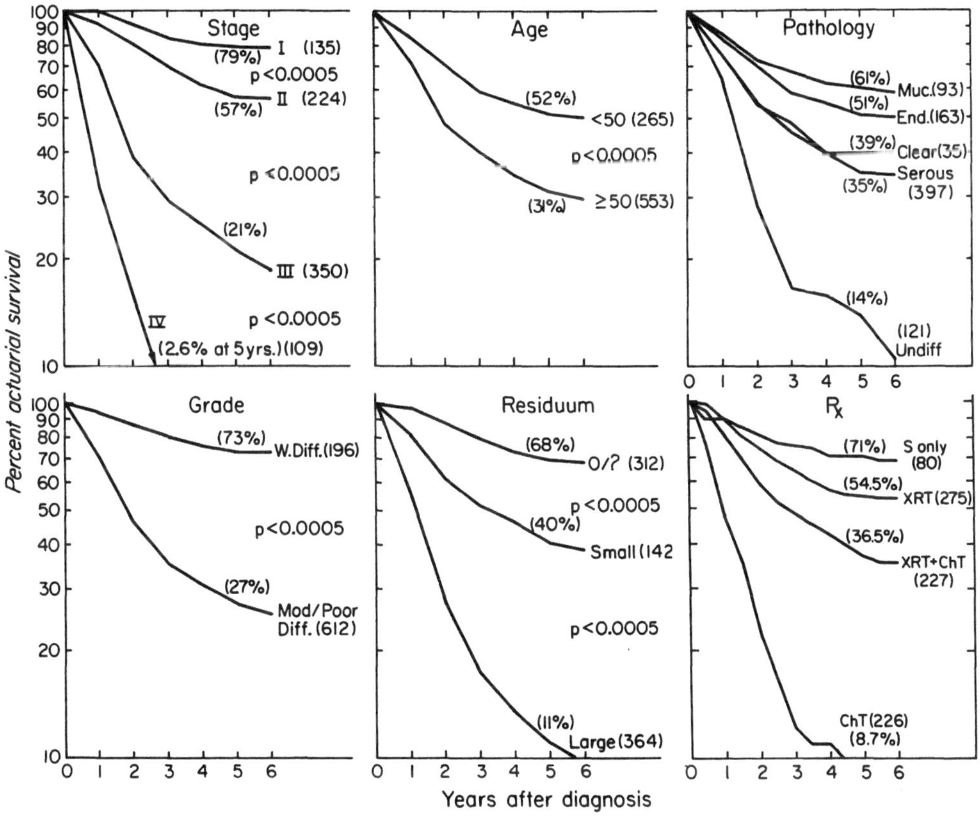

Fig. 5. The actuarial survival for various prognostic factors in 808 patients eligible for prospective trials between April 1971 and September 1978 at the PMH. Therapy: S, surgery; XRT, X-ray therapy; ChT, chemotherapy

It is clear from an examination of Fig. 5 that classifying patients according to each of the prognostic factors provides a prediction of outcome. Nevertheless, examining each prognostic factor by a univariate approach does not allow the evaluation of that prognostic factor separately from the others. That point is obvious immediately when examining the survival of patients in the different therapeutic categories. For instance, the subpopulation of patients treated by surgery alone is unlikely to be the same with respect to stage and post-operative residuum as those in the other therapeutic subgroups. Consequently, a univariate comparison does not allow the examination of each of the factors independently of any underlying prognostic differences in the populations of patients.

FIGO in their reporting of results from centres around the world have been using for several years a statistical technique to screen for the predictors that have the most influence on the 5-year survival. Bjorkholm and associates (1982) at the Radiumhemmet in Stockholm have used the same approach. They reported the independent variables which were significant in a group of 2266 patients seen between 1958 and 1973. They used death from disease as the end-point for the analysis. The independent prognostic factors which they established were clinical stage, borderline versus true malignancy, age at diagnosis, histopathological type, and extent of surgery. Combinations of these variables gave as end results subgroups whose 5-year survival rates ranged from 4% to 99%. Treatment method could not be shown to have any significant influence on survival except in advanced stages, where the extent of surgery was significant. The authors believe this finding simply reflected the extent of disease.

Although the statistical approach used by Bjorkholm and associates (1982) does help to define subgroups with dissimilar outcomes, it is not clear to me how it directly helps medical decision-making, particularly as treatment effects could not be seen. If clinical trials were carried out using stratification by the prognostic groups which have been recognised from the retrospective analysis, then there would be an improved ability to see any true difference between treatments. This is because the design would have accounted for the underlying variation due to the prognostic factors.

We have used a log-rank retrospective stratification to examine each factor independently of all others (Peto et al. 1977). Using this method, technique, stage, postoperative residuum, pathology, grade and treatment are each found to be highly significant prognostic factors. Age is also found to be significant when survival is used as the end-point of analysis, but not when relapse is used. This is most probably due to the increased risk of intercurrent death in the older age group, or less effective treatment of relapse (Dembo et al. 1982). Thus, age will not be considered as an independent prognostic factor later when relapse rates are used to establish compound prognostic groups.

After this brief discussion on individual prognostic factors, how the effect of any one may be influenced by the effect of the others, and how those that are independently significant have been established, I will present the evidence for the use of these factors in a multifactorial way. I will start with the use of just two of the prognostic factors: stage and post-operative residuum.

Prognostic Groups Using Stage Solidus Residuum

The 5-year survival for patients treated at the PMH since 1971 is 39% and compares favourably with our earlier experience of 30%. We recognised some years ago that the population of patients could be divided into two prognostic subgroups on the basis of stage and post-operative residuum (Fig. 6):

1. A poor prognosis group. These patients are rarely if ever cured by our current therapeutic approaches. They comprise approximately 45% of the total population.
2. A good prognosis group. With the previous PMH treatment strategies these patients have a 5-year survival rate of 61% with a long-term survival consistent with cure.

The attributes of stage and residuum characterising each subgroup are shown in Fig. 6. The poor prognosis group comprises patients who present with stage IV disease, or stages II and III with large residual masses following initial surgery. The 5-year survival is approximately 10%, but at 5 years the curve is still decreasing rapidly, indicating that only a few, if any, of these patients will have been cured. Neither radiation therapy nor a variety of single-agent and combination chemotherapy has demonstrated any evidence for cure, although chemotherapy is our choice for palliation.

The good prognosis patients have been characterised by stage I, II or III with no clinical evidence of disease, or stages II and III with a bilateral salpingo-oophorectomy and hysterectomy completed (comp. BSOH) even if there was residuum. Although 61% survive 5 years, the question has to be asked whether a better characterisation would help to separate those with a higher or lower chance of long-term survival. With this as an objective, I will examine next the significance of pathology and grade as it has been analysed at the PMH (Dembo et al. 1982; Dembo and Bush 1983).

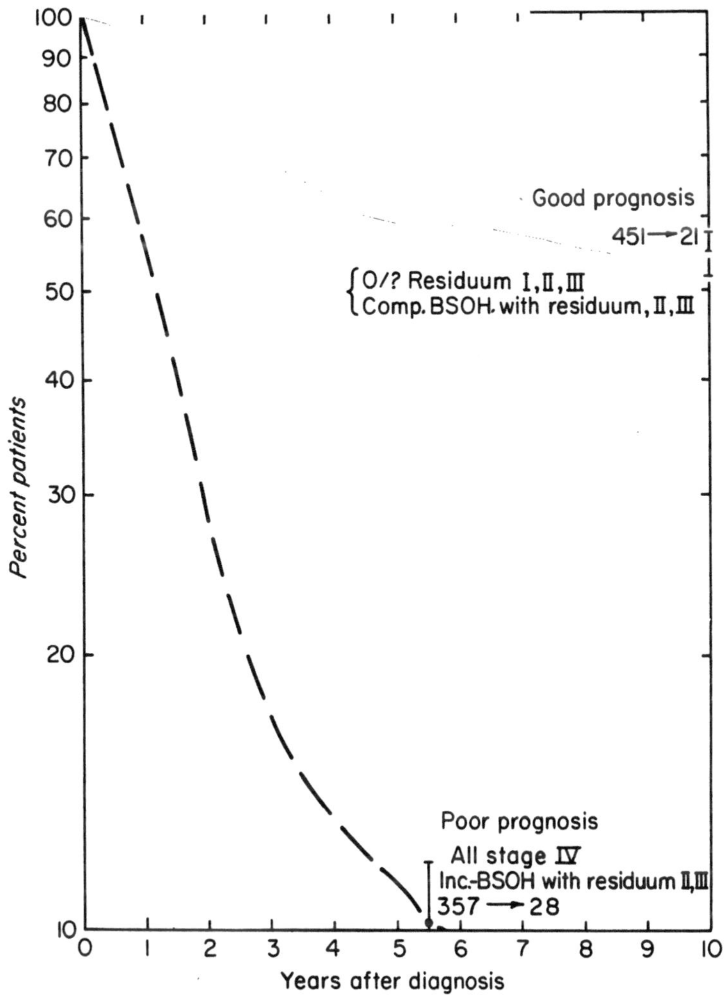

Fig. 6. The actuarial survival of the two major prognostic groupings of patients with cancer of the ovary. BSOH, bilateral salpingo-oophorectomy + hysterectomy

Prognostic Groups Using Pathology Solidus Grade

Grade of malignancy has been found to be very important prognostically, especially the recognition and classification of patients who have tumours of low potential malignancy. These are tumours in which the cellular atypia indicates cancer but no stromal invasion can be identified. Survival is excellent even in the presence of extensive and bulky disease. There is general but not universal agreement that patients with tumours classified as being of borderline malignancy should not be included in the reports of management studies of patients with invasive disease. If patients with such tumours are included, they will preferentially influence the overall survival of that population. No such patient is included in the PMH data.

There are several different pathological types within the overall classification of epithelial cancer of the ovary. As shown in Fig. 6, there are survival differences between these pathological types and also between grades.

When histological subtype and grade were examined for independence from each other, considerable variation was found in the prognostic significance of grade within the different subtypes as well as between the subtypes themselves (Dembo et al. 1982). This led to the formation of three pathology-grade subgroups within the 451 good prognosis patients as follows:

1. Serous, clear cell, well-differentiated cancer (100 patients)
2. Mucinous, endometrioid cancer; all grades (121 patients)
3. Serous, clear cell, moderately or poorly differentiated cancers, and those classified as undifferentiated (230 patients)

The 5-year survival is significantly different ($p < 0.0005$) for each subgroup, being 82% for (1), 55% for (2), and 20% for (3). The use of pathology grade subgroups for our patients appears to provide a clearer separation of high, intermediate and low survival than grade alone, although the use of the latter to form prognostic groups has been proposed by Schray et al. (1983), and is the approach used in the FIGO analysis.

Prognostic Groups Using Stage/Residuum and Pathology/Grade

When the pathology grade, residuum and stage subgroups were examined by log-rank analysis, all appeared to be independent prognostic factors. How then can a knowledge of these factors be used to assist in medical decision-making? In the literature, choice of treatment is frequently based on stage and/or residuum only. If it were possible to bring the pathology-grade information into that decision-making, treatment might be brought closer to optimal.

Table 1 shows a multifactorial grouping of patients by stage, residuum and pathology-grade of patients in the good prognosis subgroup who have been treated with post-

Table 1. A multifactorial classification of patients in the good prognosis group into three subgroups with different prognosis. WD, well differentiated; PD, poorly differentiated

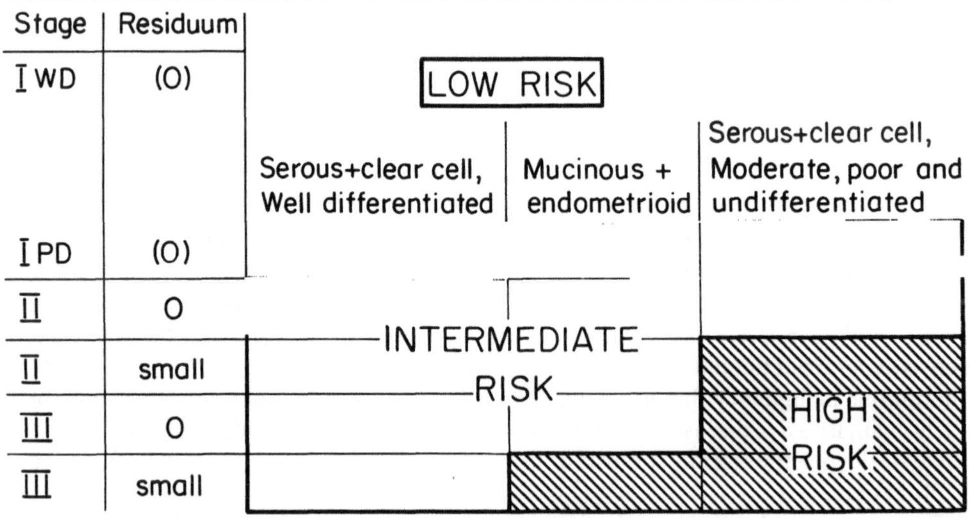

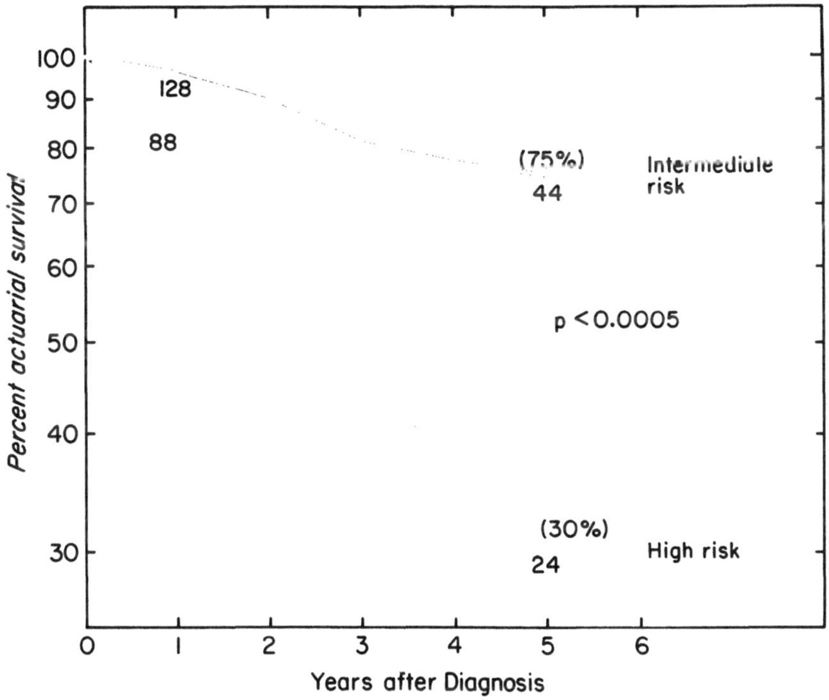

Fig. 7. The actuarial survival of patients classified as intermediate risk or high risk who have been treated with pelvic and abdomino-pelvic irradiation only

operative radiation therapy only (Dembo et al. 1982; Dembo and Bush 1983; Dembo 1983). Patients with stage I, well-differentiated cancer are at a very low risk of failure following surgery alone. Such patients will form a group which we have classified as low risk.

The remaining patients within the good prognosis group, when classified by each of the attributes shown, can be divided into two subgroups as indicated by the open and hatched areas of the table. Two-thirds of the patients fall within the open area and approximately one-third of them have relapsed since their treatment. We have classed these patients as Intermediate Risk. The remaining one-third of patients, designated by the hatched area in the table, are classed as high risk because 80% have relapsed, although 20% have remained relapse-free in the long-term.

The survival of the intermediate risk and high risk patients is shown in Fig. 7. In the intermediate risk group 75% survive in the long term, but the high risk group demonstrates only a 30% survival at 5 years, and it is to be expected that in the long term this will approach the 20% relapse-free survival for this group. Clearly improved management methods are required for this high risk group, and it is for these patients we are investigating the use of chemotherapy followed by abdomino-pelvic irradiation. Those in the intermediate risk group are being studied to determine whether there is an advantage in using a higher radiation dose than in the previous trials.

The high risk and intermediate risk subgroupings shown in Fig. 7 might differ for radiation therapy and chemotherapy, but to my knowledge no data from patients treated by chemotherapy are available to enable analysis in this multifactorial manner. More precise information on site and size of tumour residuum, and improved grading criteria, might also improve the quality of the subgroupings of patients. Also, this classification might be improved by adding information obtained from an analysis of whether a malignancy is made of cells which are diploid or aneuploid (Friedlander et al. 1983). As this type of analysis can be made from cells obtained from paraffin blocks, fresh tissue is not always necessary (Hedley et al. 1983).

Biological Speculations

Does the grouping of patients in Table 1 have any biological significance? I think it may, although direct data are not available. In the left-hand columns of the table, increasing stage and bulk are highly likely to be describing indirectly the probability of an increase in the number of residual tumour cells capable of causing relapse. Those with the least risk will be those patients with stage I disease following surgery, and those with the probability of having the highest number of cells will be those who were stage III and have clear evidence of residuum at the completion of surgery.

The pathology grade subgroups are probably describing a similar type of risk. There is increasing experimental evidence to support a model of tumour growth which is based on a concept of tumour stem cells. These are defined as the only cells in a tumour with sufficient proliferative potential to give rise to a new tumour. Such cells may divide and give rise to more stem cells or to cells committed to a differentiated pathway. In the latter case, there is evidence that proliferation becomes limited and the end stage of the differentiated pathway is sterility (MacKillop et al. 1983). Well-differentiated cancers wuld be expected to have a small proportion of tumour stem cells and a large fraction of differentiating and differentiated tumour cells. Poorly differentiated malignancies, on the other hand, would be expected to have a much higher proportion of tumour stem cells.

As this model appears appropriate for ovarian malignancies, it suggests that, as one moves from serous and clear cell well-differentiated cancers on the left-hand side of Table 1 to the poorly differentiated or undifferentiated cancers on the right, there would be an increased proportion of tumour stem cells in any residual disease. Consequently, the top left-hand corner of the table would represent the attributes associated with the smallest number of residual tumour stem cells. The bottom right-hand corner would be associated with the greatest number of tumour stem cells, both on the basis of stage-bulk and pathology-grade.

For a particular technique of radiation therapy, where the dose fractionation and anatomical volume are standard, the risk of relapse would be least for those in the top left-hand corner and greatest in the bottom right-hand corner. This is based on the assumption, and laboratory evidence, that all mammalian cells have approximately the same radiation sensitivity. Nevertheless, with increasing tumour bulk the risk of hypoxia may also increase the probability of relapse in those who meet the attributes of the lower right.

For chemotherapy, the expectation for risk of relapse is not known. If there is no major differential sensitivity between tumour types and grade, then similar risks of relapse to that following radiation would be expected for the same number of treatments. If the Goldie-Coldman model is correct (Goldie and Coldman 1979), there may be a decreased probability of resistant populations being present as one moves from well-differentiated to the poorly or undifferentiated carcinomas. This is because the latter have a higher proportion of stem cells, a consequent smaller total number of stem cell divisions in the history of the malignancy, and thus a lower probability of having developed chemotherapy-resistant subpopulations. Such a model would lend support to the use in those patients on the right-hand side of Table 1 of chemotherapy or chemotherapy combined with radiation rather than a higher dose of radiation.

Summary and Conclusions

This review of the use of radiation in the management of patients with ovarian cancer has tried to provide sufficient information to answer the questions posed at the beginning of the discussion. These were:

What role does radiation therapy have that currently cannot be replaced by any other modality?

I have presented evidence that radiation therapy does have a curative role, particularly in those patients classified by stage, post-operative residuum, grade and pathology as an intermediate risk subgroup. Their 5-year survival is estimated at 75% using past PMH radiation techniques. For such patients there is no evidence yet in the literature to show that chemotherapy provides the same opportunity for long-term survival. To put the intermediate risk patients into a perspective with the rest of the population, the proposed categorisation of patients for management purposes will be given and is as follows:

1. *Poor prognosis patients:* These are approximately 45% of the population. Treatment is mainly palliative, but with the use of cisplatin in chemotherapeutic combinations a much higher response rate has been realised than previously. This has led to an increase in median survival although there is no evidence yet of any increase in the proportion with long-term survival. Nevertheless, the improved response rates raise hope that by adding either abdomino-pelvic radiation or other combinations of drugs, some improvement in long-term survival may be achieved. Only 10% survive 5 years, and fewer than this in the longer term.
2. *Good prognosis patients:* These make up 55% of the total population but can be subdivided into three prognostic subgroups by multifactorial methods.
   a) *Low risk:* These are approximately 5% of the total population. They have a very high survival (>95%) following surgery alone.
   b) *Intermediate risk:* These comprise about 33% of the population. Using abdomino-pelvic radiation with a pelvic boost approximately 75% survive in the long term.
   c) *High risk:* These patients make up approximately 17% of the population. With radiation therapy only 20% survive relapse free, and improved methods of management are required.

The survival for the total population following the above strategy would be expected to be 38%-40%, although the generally accepted overall survival for patients with cancer of the ovary is 30%-33%.

How important are other modalities in ensuring that the maximum benefit and minimum toxicity are achieved from the use of radiation therapy?

There is evidence indicating that those patients with zero or minimal post-operative residuum are benefited most by adjuvant or adjunctive therapy, and that by further resection surgery can favourably influence survival. Nevertheless, it is still not clear how many patients can be benefited, and in how many cases the ability to resect completely is an indication of the nature of the disease.

Are there physical or biological mechanisms which can explain success or failure in the survival advantage demonstrated for radiation therapy?

Radiation techniques which encompass the whole peritoneal cavity produce higher survival rates and fewer relapses than those which treat only part of the abdomen. Anatomical volume has to be considered as a higher priority than radiation dose. From the multifactorial prognostic groups formed to help select those patients appropriately treated with abdomino-pelvic irradiation it is possible to theorise about possible biological mechanisms; in particular, whether the prognostic groups indicate groups of patients with a differing total number of tumour stem cells which have to be sterilised before cure can be achieved.

I hope that I have also demonstrated that building each new trial on the basis of a preceding trial allows both an approach to optimising treatment, and the development of a detailed data base which allows the generation of hypotheses that can be used to design the next trial. It must also be clear from this discussion that the greatest challenge comes from the large proportion of patients who present with extensive bulky disease. Although new approaches to management have been discussed, to meet this challenge most successfully may require a major programme to examine the epidemiology, the improvement of screening and methods for early diagnosis, together with a better understanding of the biology of ovarian cancer.

References

American Cancer Society (1983) Ca, Cancer Journal for Clinicians. New York, Vol 33, No 1

Bagley CM, Young RC, Canellos GP, DeVita VT (1972) Treatment of ovarian carcinoma: Possibilities for progress. New Engl J Med 278: 856-862

Bagley CM Jr, Young RC, Schein PS, Chabner BA, DeVita VT (1973) Ovarian carcinoma metastatic to the diaphragm: Frequently undiagnosed at laparotomy. A preliminary report. Am J Obstet Gynecol 116: 397

Bell DR, Woods RL, Levi JA, Fox RM, Tattersall MHN (1982) Advanced ovarian cancer: a prospective randomized trial of chlorambucil versus combined cyclophosphamide and *cis*-diamminedichloroplatinum. Aust NZ J Med 12: 245-249

Bjorkholm E, Pettersson F, Einhorn N, Breds I, Bilsson B, Tjernberg B (1982) Long-term follow-up and prognostic factors in ovarian carcinoma. Acta Radiol Oncol 21: 413-419

Bush RS (1979a) Malignancies of the ovary, uterus and cervix. Edward Arnold, London, p 34

Bush RS (1979b) Editorial: Problems related to the evaluation of reported results in cancer of the ovary. Int J Radiat Oncol Biol Phys 5: 2157-2160

Bush RS (1984) The contribution of radiation therapy to the management of patients with cancer of the ovary. Arthur W. Erskine Lecture. Radiology (in press)

Bush RS, Dembo AJ (1980) Current status of treatment for patients with ovarian cancer. In: CE Newman, CJH Ford, JA Jordan (eds) Ovarian cancer. Advances in the biosciences vol 26. Pergamon Press, Oxford, pp 115-134

Bush RS, Dembo AJ (1984) Radiation therapy for patients with ovarian cancer. In: CN Hudson (ed) Ovarian cancer. Oxford University Press (in press)

Bush RS, Allt WEC, Beale FA, Bean HA, Pringle JF, Sturgeon J (1977) Treatment of epithelial carcinoma of the ovary: Operation, irradiation and chemotherapy. Am J Obstet Gynecol 127: 692-704

Bush RS, DeBoer G, Hill RP (1982) Long term survival with gynecological cancer. In: BA Stoll (ed) Prolonged arrest in cancer. New targets in cancer treatment vol 1. Wiley, New York, pp 27-57

Ciampi A, Till JE (1980) Null results in clinical trials: The need for a decision-theory approach. Br J Cancer 41: 618-628

Clarke EA (1983) Head, Ontario Cancer Registry. Personel communication

Delclos L, Quinlan EJ (1969) Malignant tumors of the ovary managed with post-operative megavoltage irradiation. Radiology 93: 659

Delclos L, Dembo AJ (1980) Ovaries. In: GH Fletcher (ed) Textbook of radiotherapy. Lea and Febiger, Philadelphia, pp 834-951

Dembo AJ (1983) Radiation therapy in the management of ovarian cancer. Clin Obstet Gynecol 10: 261-278

Dembo AJ, Bush RS (1983) Radiation therapy of ovarian carcinoma. In: CT Griffiths, AF Fuller (eds) Gynecologic oncology. Martinus Nijhoff, Boston, pp 262-298

Dembo AJ, Bush RS, Beale FA, Bean HA, Pringle JA, Sturgeon J (1979 a) The Princess Margaret Hospital study of ovarian cancer: Stages I, II and asymptomatic III presentation. Cancer Treat Rep 62: 249-254

Dembo AJ, VanDyk J, Japp B, Bean HA, Beale FA, Pringle JF, Bush RS (1979 b) Whole abdominal irradiation by a moving-strip technique for patients with ovarian cancer. Int J Radiat Oncol Biol Phys 5: 1933-1942

Dembo AJ, Bush RS, DeBoer G (1981) Letter to the editor. Am J Obstet Gynecol 141: 231

Dembo AJ, Bush RS, Brown TC (1982) Clinico-pathological correlates in ovarian cancer. Bull Cancer (Paris) 69: 292-297

Dembo AJ, Bush RS, Beale FA, Bean HA, Fine S, Gospodarowicz M, Herman J, Pringle JF, Sturgeon J, Thomas GM (1983) A randomized clinical trial of moving strip versus open field whole abdominal irradiation in patients with invasive epithelial cancer of the ovary. Proc Am Soc Clin Oncol 2: Abstr C-571

Feldman GB, Knapp RC (1974) Lymphatic drainage of the peritoneal cavity and its significance in ovarian cancer. Am J Obstet Gynecol 119: 991

Friedlander ML, Taylor IW, Russell P, Musgrove EA, Hedley DW, Tattersall MHN (1983) Ploidy as a prognostic factor in ovarian cancer. Int J Gynecol Pathol 2: 55-63

Fuks Z, Rizel S, Anteby SO, Biran S (1982) The multimodal approach to the treatment of Stage III ovarian carcinoma. Int J Radiat Oncol Biol Phys 8: 903-908

Goldie JH, Coldman AJ (1979) A mathematical model for relating the drug sensitivity of tumours to their spontaneous mutation rate. Cancer Treat Rep 63: 1727-1733

Griffiths CT, Parker LM, Fuller AF (1970) Role of cytoreductive surgical treatment in the management of advanced ovarian cancer. Cancer Treat Rep 63: 235-240

Haas JS, Mansfield CM, Hartman GV et al. (1980) Results of radiation therapy in the treatment of epithelial carcinoma of the ovary. Cancer 46: 1950

Hainsworth JD, Malcolm A, Johnson DH, Burnett LS, Jones III HW, Greco FA (1983) Advanced minimal residual ovarian carcinoma: abdominopelvic irradiation following combination chemotherapy. Obstet Gynecol 61: 619-623

Hedley DW, Friedlander ML, Taylor IW, Rugg CA, Musgrove EA (1983) Method for analysis of cellular DNA content of paraffin-embedded pathological material using flow cytometry. J Histochem Cytochem 31: 1333-1335

Hreshchyshyn MM, Park RC, Blessing JA, Norris HJ, Levy D, Lagasse LD, Creasman WT (1980) The role of adjuvant therapy in Stage I ovarian cancer. Am J Obstet Gynecol 138: 139-145

Kottmeier HL (ed) (1979) Annual report on the results of treatment in gynecological cancer vol 17 1969-1972. International Federation of Gynecology and Obstetrics Stockholm
Lewis GC, Blessing J (1977) Ovarian cancer: Use of multiple modality programs involving surgery, radiation therapy and chemotherapy. Cancer 40: 588-594
MacKillop WJ, Ciampi A, Till JE, Buick RN (1983) A stem cell model of human tumour growth: implications for tumor cell clonogenic assays. J Natl Cancer Inst 70: 9-16
Peto R, Pike MC, Armitage P, Breslow NE, Cox DR, Howard SV, Martel N, McPherson K, Petro J, Smith PG (1977) Design and analysis of randomized clinical trials requiring prolonged observation of each patient. II. Analysis and example. Br J Cancer 35: 1-39
Registrar General of Ontario (1978) Vital Statistics for 1978, Province of Ontario
Rosenshein NB, Leichner PK, Vogelsang G (1979) Radiocolloids in the treatment of ovarian cancer. Obstet Gynecol Survey 34: 708-720
Santesson L, Kottmeier HL (1968) Ovarian cancer. UICC Monograph Series, vol 11. Springer-Verlag, Berlin Heidelberg New York, p 1
Schray M, Martinez A, Cox R, Ballon S (1983) Radiotherapy in epithelial ovarian cancer: Analysis of prognostic factors based on long-term experience. Obstet Gynecol 62: 373-382
Schwartz PE, Smith JP (1980) Second-look operations in ovarian cancer. Am J Obstet Gynecol 18: 1124-1130
Scully RE (1970) Recent progress in ovarian cancer. Hum Pathol 1: 73-98
Smith JP (1980) Surgery for ovarian cancer. In: CE Newman, CJH Ford, JA Jordan (eds) Ovarian cancer. Advances in the biosciences, vol 26. Pergamon Press, Oxford, pp 115-134
Smith JP, Rutledge F (1970) Chemotherapy in the treatment of cancer of the ovary. Am J Obstet Gynecol 107: 691-703
Smith JP, Rutledge FN, Delclos L (1975) Postoperative treatment of early cancer of the ovary: A random trial between postoperative irradiation and chemotherapy. Natl Cancer Inst Monogr 52: 149-153
Sturgeon JFG, Fine S, Gospodarowicz MK, Dembo AJ, Bean HA, Bush RS, Beale FA, Herman JG, Pringle JF, Thomas GM (1981) A randomized trial of melphalan alone versus combination chemotherapy in advanced ovarian cancer. Proc Soc Gynecol Oncol: abstr 28:

The Usefulness of the Human Tumour Stem Cell Assay

C. J. Williams

CRC Medical Oncology Unit, Centre Block CF99, Southampton General Hospital, Tremona Road, Southampton S09 4XY, United Kingdom

For the past 30 years alkylating agents have formed the backbone of chemotherapy for advanced ovarian carcinoma. Up to a half of patients so treated show a useful response, but prolonged remissions are uncommon. More recently a variety of additional drugs with similar orders of activity have become available (Table 1). Current randomised studies comparing combinations of empirically chosen drugs with a single alkylating agent have failed to show a survival advantage for the combination (Omura et al. 1983; Carmo-Pereira 1983; Bruckner et al. 1983; Vogl et al. 1983; Williams et al. 1983 a). Many current combinations have contained cisplatin (Williams et al. 1982) and because of this are highly toxic. Chemotherapy, therefore, continues to make little impact on the survival of patients with less than optimal initial surgery despite the high remission rates achieved with current combinations (Table 2).

More active cytotoxic chemotherapy will be needed if there are to be improvements in the outlook for the large number of women who have advanced ovarian carcinoma. There are two possible approaches using cytotoxic drugs: one is to try to use current agents in better ways, the other is to develop new and more effective drugs. Currently drugs are selected for combination chemotherapy according to empirical rules. The availability of an in vitro assay for the selection of the most active drugs in an individual patient's tumour could be one way of developing more effective combinations of drugs already available.

Table 1. Objective response rates for single agents in advanced ovarian cancer

Drug	No. of patients	Objective response rate (%)
Alkylating agents		
Melphalan	541	47
Cyclophosphamide	335	43
Chlorambucil	388	51
Triethylenethiophosphoramide	337	48
Nitrosoureas	48	13
Non-alkylating agents		
Cisplatin	304	33
Hexamethylmelamine	108	35
Adriamycin	108	20
Methotrexate	37	30
5-Fluorouracil	116	20

After Tobias and Griffiths (1976)

Ovarian Cancer, Ed. by N. M. Bleehen

Table 2. Activity of platinum-based drug combinations in unrandomised studies

Author	No. of patients	Overall response rate (%)	Median survival (months)	Drugs[a]
Vogl et al. (ECOG) (1983)	38	93	24	Cisplatin, cyclo, adria, HXM
Holland et al. (1981)	48	73	20	Cisplatin, adria, HXM
Erlich (1979)	56	78	24	Cisplatin, cyclo, adria
Williams et al. (1982)	35	80	19	Cisplatin, cyclo, adria

[a] Cyclo, cyclophosphamide; adria, adriamycin (doxorubicin); HXM, hexamethylmelamine

Such an assay could also be used greatly to speed up and improve the accuracy of selection of new drugs for clinical trial.

Although there have been many in vitro predictive tests for cancer chemotherapy (Mattern and Volm 1982) the human tumour stem cell assay (HTSCA) or clonogenic assay first described by Hamburger and Salmon (1977) has received most attention in the past 5 years. This chapter reviews critically the current usefulness of this assay in epithelial ovarian cancer.

Concept Behind Clonogenic Assays

The growth properties of populations of neoplastic cells are in agreement with a model in which cells with a proliferative potential form a continuum of a mixture of cells some of which are without ability or have only limited ability to divide while others have a capacity to renew themselves (Mendelsohn and Dethlefsen 1968; Steel 1977). The self-renewing and population-renewing cells, called stem cells, may only form a small part of the total tumour population, but are responsible for tumour repopulation after treatment and for metastatic growth. These cells are, therefore, the likely primary target of any anti-cancer chemotherapy.

Assessment of the effectiveness of treatment on an unselected tumour cell population may be misleading as important effects on the small number of stem cells can be skewed by a lack of effect on the large number of non-stem cells. Assessment of treatment effect on stem cells must measure their capacity to continue to reproduce and form colonies of cells: in other words it must be a clonogenic assay. However, it must be remembered that short-term colony formation by itself may not be a sufficient test of effect on stem cells; transitional cells can form small colonies (Selby et al. 1983).

Outline of the Method for the HTSC Assay (Hamburger and Salmon 1977; Hamburger et al. 1978; Salmon et al. 1978; Von Hoff et al. 1981 a)

Viable tumour cells must be obtained from the patient; this may be from malignant effusions or solid tumours. Ideally they should be processed as soon as possible because delay reduces viability. The cells must be disaggregated to a single-cell suspension; this is prerequisite of the assay. If a drug assay is performed the cells are exposed to various concentrations of the specific drug under test; in most studies this has been for 1 h at 37 °C, though some workers have used continuous exposure. Cells are then plated in 0.3% molten agar above a 0.5% agar feeder layer, incubated at 37 °C in a humidified 7.5% carbon dioxide atmosphere and watched for colony growth.

Technical Problems

Difficulty in Preparing a Single-cell Suspension

In the original descriptions of the assay, mechanical methods were used to disaggregate solid tumours. More recently, studies which have compared enzymatic methods with mechanical means have shown that enzymes yield better results (Slocum et al. 1981; Hamburger et al. 1982; Morgan et al. 1983). However, despite improved methods of disaggregation it is difficult to exclude all clumps. It should be remembered that one clump per 1000 cells, if mistaken for a colony, would yield a plating efficiency of 0.1%, which is well within the normal range.

Colony Size

Most current studies define a colony as being made up of 30 to 50 or more cells. However, transitional cells may give rise to small colonies, which may lead to an over-estimation of cell survival. It has been suggested that one way round this problem could be that the distribution of colonies by size may be used to separate those derived from stem cells from those derived from transitional cells (MacKillop et al. 1983).

Number of Tumours Suitable for Drug Assay

Plating efficiencies are very low with this assay, but in order to compare colony formation in drug-exposed cells and control cells a minimum of 30–50 colonies are required in the control plate. In most studies the number of tumours forming more than 50 colonies is low (<50%) and a drug sensitivity assay cannot be performed for these tumours (Von Hoff et al. 1981 a, 1982). In the earlier and larger of the studies by Von Hoff's group (1981 a) only 199 of 800 tumours (25%) formed more than 30 colonies, whilst in the subsequent study (1982) 58% of 604 specimens yielded more than 30 colonies. Overall Von Hoff's group have cultured more than 8000 tumours, of which only 31% showed sufficient growth in vitro for tumour testing. Perhaps more importantly only 8% with adequate growth showed in vitro sensitivity to available anti-cancer drugs (Von Hoff 1983). The clinical applicability of the assay depends on tumour type, method of collection and technique of the assay.

Table 3. Clonogenicity of human ovarian tumours and principal reasons for rejection from the study of Bertoncello et al. (1982)

Reason for rejection	No. of biopsies	Solid tumours	Effusions
Low cellularity	22	3	19
Low viability	14	12	2
Aggregations	12	1	11
Tumour histology/cytology negative	12	1	11
Indefinite histology/cytology	3	0	3
Contamination	3	3	0
Insufficient tumour	7	5	2
Total rejected	73	25	48
Amenable to assay	41 (36%)	16 (39%)	25 (34%)
Total	114	41	73

Table 4. Clonogenicity of human breast cancer according to hormone receptor status

Cytosolic oestrogen receptor status	No. of tumour samples tested	No. forming colonies (%)[a]
Positive	23	5[b] (22)
Negative	21	14 (67) ($p < 0.01$)

[a] Colony growth defined as more than five colonies of at least 30 cells
[b] None of the five receptor-positive colonies which grew was nuclear receptor positive

Currently it would appear that in only 25%-50% of cases will there be sufficient colonies to perform a drug assay and only a minor proportion of these assays will show in vitro drug sensitivity. The difficulties in performing this assay are underlined by the finding of Bertoncello et al. (1982) that only 41 (36%) out of 114 specimens of ovarian carcinoma formed colonies. Reasons for rejection of tumour specimens in this study are shown in Table 3.

Tumour Biology and Possible Growth Factors

Although it should be possible to grow all tumours in a culture system, many individual tumours do not grow well in this assay and certain tumour types are much more difficult than others. In a study of breast cancer (Williams et al. 1983b; Smallwood et al. 1984) cells from tumours possessing oestrogen hormone receptors grew significantly less well than those without oestrogen receptors (Table 4). This correlation did not appear to be due to an inherent kinetic advantage since the thymidine labelling index of receptor-positive tumours growing was similar to that of the receptor-negative group. It seems most likely that the culture method selects for the growth of receptor-negative tumours or lacks the necessary growth factors needed by receptor-positive tumours. Such biological differences need to be investigated before potential clinical applications in a wide variety of tumours can be fulfilled. Already a number of growth factors have been identified and attempts made to develop serum-free media (Calvo et al. 1983; Barnes and Sato 1980a, b; Carney et al. 1981), but optimum conditions will undoubtedly vary from tumour to tumour. The effect of the presence of autologous phagocytic cells which increase colony formation has also been investigated (Hamburger et al. 1983). Uitendaal et al. (1983) have shown that enriched CMRL 1066 medium used in the assay can be replaced by cell-free ascites from tumour patients and that this enhances colony formation.

Analysis of Data

Many of the published drug sensitivity curves are based on very few points because of the difficulty in performing these assays. Selby and Steel (1982) have questioned whether the plateaus seen in many in vitro sensitivity curves may be unrepresentative of the sensitivity of treatment in vivo. The method used to correlate in vitro and in vivo results can be expressed in several different ways and the apparent usefulness of the test influenced by the incidence of positive and negative clinical results. For instance the accurate in vitro prediction of resistance in 90% of cases is less impressive if 90% of the tumours are resistant in vivo. Unfortunately, this has been the case in many of the previously treated patients in current series.

Method of Drug Exposure

In vitro exposure of tumour cells to drugs is unlikely to represent the pharmacological effects of the drug when given to a patient. Although attempts have been made to use concentrations achievable in patients' plasma (Alberts and Chen 1980), these concentrations are unlikely to be analogous to those achieved in a tumour. The use of 1-h incubations or continuous exposure are similarly not representative of in vivo pharmacokinetics. Drug metabolism is altered and some drugs such as cyclophosphamide need bioactivation (Colvin and Hilton 1981).

Combinations

Nearly all studies of sensitivity have used single drugs, although most patients with cancer receive a combination of drugs. The only valid way of testing for synergy and antagonism is to use the method of isobolograms (Berenbaum 1977). However, this requires the use of multiple dose levels of each drug, and obtaining enough cells for assays of a single drug is already a major problem. No acceptable method for evaluating combinations is therefore currently available.

Results of HTSC Assay in Ovarian Carcinoma

Having outlined some of the potential difficulties of the assay system, the question needs to be asked as to what progress has been made in the specific case of ovarian carcinoma. Fortunately this tumour is more easily grown in the assay system than most tumours and

Table 5. Growth rates for ovarian carcinoma using the human tumour stem cell assay

Tumour source	No. plated	No. grown (%)[a]
Solid tumour	92	85 (92)
Effusion	57	54 (95)
Total	149	139 (93)

After Welander and Alberts (1985)
[a] Growth is defined as ⩾30 colonies per control plate and enough cells to perform at least one drug assay

Table 6. Drug sensitivity in the human tumour stem cell assay for ovarian carcinoma

Drug	Historical clinical response rate (%)	No. of assays	No. sensitive or intermediate (%)[a]	No. resistant (%)
Doxorubicin[b]	20	70	11 (16)	59 (84)
Cisplatin[b]	39	71	12 (17)	59 (83)
5-Fluorouracil[b]	20	99	46 (47)	53 (54)
Vinblastine[b]	12	69	20 (29)	49 (71)
Vincristine[c]	0	90	28 (31)	62 (69)
Mitomycin[d]	20	61	21 (34)	40 (66)

[a] Sensitivity is defined as colony survival below 30% of control using drug concentration one-tenth of achievable peak plasma level. Intermediate sensitivity is 31%–50% colony survival
[b] After Welander and Alberts (1984) Griffiths (1982); [c] Wasserman et al. (1975); [d] Crooke (1979)

some series have reported high rates of colony formation. Welander (Welander and Alberts 1985) was able to grow over 90% of the tumours they received (Table 5). Bertoncello et al. (1982), in contrast, successfully grew only 36% of the specimens they received.

Individual anti-cancer drugs have been tested on previously untreated tumour cells in the assay system and the results then compared with response rates previously reported in phase II trials (Table 6). In the study by Welander et al. (1983) some drugs used clinically for second-line treatment appeared more active in the assay than those used as primary therapy. These types of data, whilst of interest, are so dependent on variables such as clinical dose and schedule and the reliability of the in vitro method of drug exposure, that little can yet be made of them.

Whilst many of the same problems apply, a more useful test of the results of in vitro tumour sensitivity tests is the direct correlation of in vitro and in vivo responses in a prospective trial. Welander and Alberts (1985) have reported on sensitivity patterns in a prospective study of 50 previously untreated patients and 82 who had received prior chemotherapy (Table 7). Three hundred and fifty-nine drug assays were performed for the 50 untreated patients, with only 21% showing sensitive or intermediate responses. For the 82 previously treated patients 395 assays were done, with 25% showing sensitive or intermediate responses. These low rates of in vitro sensitivity are disappointing and, if correct, suggest that ovarian carcinoma is relatively resistant to current drug therapy. These response rates are considerably lower than those seen clinically with some drugs (Table 1). The lack of increase in resistance in those previously treated also is not borne out by clinical experience in virtually any tumour. In addition, these data are in conflict with those of

Table 7. Drug sensitivity according to the human tumour stem cell assay in untreated and pre-treated patients with ovarian carcinoma

Prior treatment	No. of patients	No. of drugs tested	No. sensitive or intermediate (%)[a]	No. resistant (%)
No prior chemotherapy	50	359	77 (21)	282 (79)
Failed prior chemotherapy	82	395	99 (25)	296 (75)
Total	132	754	176 (23)	578 (77)

After Welander and Alberts (1985)
[a] Defined in Table 5

Table 8. In vitro/in vivo correlations of human tumour stem cell assay in ovarian carcinoma

Source	No. of trials	In vitro/in vivo[a]			
		S/S	S/R	R/S	R/R
Alberts (1980)	95	14	7	1	73
Natale (1981)	28	10	3	1	14
Welander	19	9	1	0	9
Total	142[b]	33	11	2	96

From Welander and Alberts (1985)
[a] R, resistant; S, sensitive
44 patients

Predictive Accuracy: sensitivity 75%; resistance 98%

Alberts et al. (1981 a), where cells from tumours previously exposed to chemotherapy were resistant - though the method of analysis of the assay results was different.

When the in vitro- and in vivo results for single agents are correlated (Table 8) the predictive accuracy for resistance is high (98%) whilst that for sensitivity is somewhat lower (75%). The data are from a relatively small number of patients (44) with apparent high accuracy of prediction of resistance. Resistance was, however, present in vivo in 74%, and moderate accuracy in predicting sensitivity cannot be used to validate the assay. Validation of the assay as a predictive tool can only come from a prospective clinical trial in which it is used to select therapy. Alberts et al. (1981 b) have reported on the survival of 37 patients who had relapsed after chemotherapy. Drug sensitivity was tested in the assay and in 22 patients active drugs were identified and patients were treated with one of these. The overall objective clinical response rate for these patients was 73% with a median survival of 12.6 months. The other 15 patients, in whom no active drug was identified by the assay, received empirically selected chemotherapy. The response rate in this group was 20% with a median survival of 4.5 months. Though it shows a large difference between the two groups, this trial contains a major bias as the group receiving empirical treatment was highly likely to be resistant to chemotherapy. The only conclusion that can be drawn is confirmation that the assay is able to identify patients unlikely to benefit from treatment.

A more objective test of the assay is to identify sensitivity patterns in previously untreated patients and then to randomise patients between drugs selected either according to the assay or to an empirical combination (Von Hoff 1983). Taking into account the difficulties experienced when using the assay and the problems of interpreting the results when combinations are used, Von Hoff (1983) suggests that well over 1000 patients would be needed in such a study. Although such studies are underway, no results are available.

Survival and Drug Sensitivity According to Clonogenicity

Some studies have shown that the aggressiveness of a tumour may be related to cloning efficiency (Mattox & Von Hoff 1980; Von Hoff et al. 1981 b; Bertoncello et al. 1982; Sutherland et al. 1983). Patients in these studies whose tumours did not form colonies relapsed less frequently than those which grew and their survival was better. Some studies have also suggested that patients whose tumour does not grow in the assay system are more likely to respond to chemotherapy (Sutherland et al. 1983). Sandbach et al. (1982) and Sutherland et al. (1983) have found, in keeping with other workers, that only a small proportion (about 15%) of tumours tested showed drug sensitivity; this is in contrast to clinical response rates of 50%–70% in tumours such as breast cancer. Sutherland and his co-workers have suggested that if low colony counts or failure to form colonies, improve the chance of having a response, the response rate in this group of patients with high colony counts (> 30) may accurately reflect a low response rate.

Heterogeneity

Tumours appear to be inherently heterogeneous (Mihich et al. 1979) and clonal heterogeneity has been found using this assay system (MacKintosh et al. 1981; Bertoncello et al. 1982). MacKintosh showed that five cell lines derived from individual agar clones grown from a single human ovarian tumour all exhibited differing patterns of growth, morphology and drug sensitivity in culture. Such heterogeneity may be a major problem when testing drugs, especially when they are used as single agents.

Screening of New Drugs

The Division of Cancer Treatment of the National Cancer Institute in the United States screens over 15000 new compounds for anti-tumour activity each year (Von Hoff et al. 1979). Most screening has used animal models such as P-388 leukaemia, though human tumour xenografts have been used recently. In the past few years the HTSC assay has been used (Von Hoff & Bradley 1979; Salmon et al. 1981) to test standard drugs and those under investigation, such as M-AMSA, ICRF187 and PALA, against patients tumours. Agents not yet used in man, such as AT125 and *cis*-retinoic acid (Meyskens and Salmon 1979) have also been tested.

Ideally new drugs should be tested in at least 14 patients with each of the major tumour types. Though it does seem possible to do this (Salmon et al. 1982) it is a major logistical exercise. Currently it appears that the assay would have identified the active drugs used at present. However, we need drugs with a different pattern of activity from those currently in use. Ideally a new model would identify drugs which would have been missed in previous assay systems, as a new assay mimicking available animal models is no advance at all. The HTSCA assay may fulfil these hopes, though this will have to await the outcome of studies of the assay as a screening tool by the National Cancer Institute.

Conclusion

Currently the human tumour stem cell assay and other predictive assays must remain a research tool. No study has conclusively shown that the choice of chemotherapy according to such an assay will improve a patient's chances of survival. Clinically the assay is being tested for use as a screening tool for new drugs (Salmon et al. 1982) and as a means of detecting small numbers of tumour cells (Pollard et al. 1981), and it may also be useful as a biological model of tumours (Salmon et al. 1982).

Much basic work is needed before we can hope to find out whether assay systems of this type will have clinical relevance. The assay remains time-consuming and cumbersome and must be improved if it is ever to be accepted into general use.

References

Alberts D, Chen H (1980) Summary of pharmacokinetic parameters relevant to in vitro drug assay. In: S. Salmon (ed) Cloning of human tumour cells. Alan Liss Inc, New York, pp 351-359

Alberts D, Chen H, Salmon S et al (1981 a) Chemotherapy of ovarian cancer directed by the human tumour stem cell assay. Cancer Chemother Pharmacol 6: 279-285

Alberts D, Chen H, Young L et al. (1981 b) Improved survival of relapsing ovarian cancer patients using the human tumour stem cell assay to select chemotherapy. Proc ASCO 22: 462 (abstr)

Barnes D, Sato G (1980 a) Serum-free cell culture: A unifying approach. Cell 22: 645-648

Barnes D, Sato G (1980 b) Methods for growth of cultured cells in serum-free medium. Analyt Biochem 102: 255-258

Berenbaum M (1977) Synergism, additivism and antagonism. In: Immunosuppression: A critical review. Clin Exp Immunol 28: 1-18

Bertoncello T, Bradley J, Campbell J, Day A, McDonald I, McLiesh G, Quinn M, Rome R, Hodgson G (1982) Limitations of the clonal agar assay for the assessment of primary human ovarian tumour biopsies. Br J Cancer 45: 803-811

Bruckner H, Cohen C, Goldberg J (1983) Cisplatin regimes and improved prognosis of patients with poorly differentiated tumours. Am J Obstet Gynecol 145: 653-658

Calvo F, Carney D, Brower M, Minna J (1983) Hormone supplemented media for cloning human breast cancer: Increased colony formation without alteration of chemosensitivity. Br J Cancer 48: 683-688

Carmå-Pereira J (1983) Cis-platinum, adriamycin and hexamethylmelamine versus cyclophosphamide in advanced ovarian carcinoma. Cancer Chemother Pharmacol 10: 100-103

Carney D, Bunn P, Gazdar A, Pagan J, Minna J (1981) Selective growth in serum-free hormone supplemented media of tumour cells obtained by biopsy from patients with small cell carcinoma of the lungs. Proc Natl Acad Sci USA 78: 3185-3187

Colvin M, Hilton J (1981) Pharmacology of cyclophosphamide and its metabolites. Cancer Treat Rep 65: 89-95

Crooke S (1979) Mitomycin C: an overview. In: S Carter, S Crooke (eds) Mitomycin C: current status and new developments. Academic Press, New York London, pp 1-20

Ehrlich C, Einhorn L, Williams S (1979) Chemotherapy for stage III-IV epithelial ovarian cancer

with cisdichlorodiammineplatinum (II), adriamycin and cyclophosphamide: A preliminary report. Cancer Treat Rep 63: 281-288
Griffiths C (1982) Carcinoma of the ovary and fallopian tube. In: J Holland, E Frei (eds) Cancer medicine. Lea and Febiger, Philadelphia, pp 1958-1972
Hamburger A, Salmon S (1977) Primary bioassay of human tumour stem cells. Science 197: 461-463
Hamburger A, Salmon S, Kim N, Trent J, Soehnlen B, Alberts D, Schmidt H (1978) Direct cloning of human ovarian carcinoma cells in agar. Cancer Res 38: 3438-3444
Hamburger A, White C, Tencer K (1982) Effect of enzymatic disaggregation on proliferation of human tumour cells in soft agar. J Natl Cancer Inst 68: 945-949
Hamburger A, White C, Dunn F (1983) Modulation of tumour colony growth by irradiated accessory cells. Br J Cancer 98: 675-682
Holland J, Bruckner H, Cohen C (1981) Cisplatin therapy of ovarian cancer. In: A Prestayko, S Cooke (eds) Cisplatin: Current status and new developments. Academic Press, New York, pp 383-391
MacKillop W, Ciampi A, Till J, Buick R (1983) A stem cell model of human tumour growth: Implications for tumour cell clonogenic assays. J Natl Cancer Inst 70: 9-16
MacKintosh M, Louie A, Evans T (1981) Clonal heterogeneity in a human ovarian carcinoma. Proc AACR 22: 379 (Abstr)
Mattern J, Volm M (1982) Clinical relevance of predictive tools for cancer chemotherapy. Cancer Treat Rev 9: 267-298
Mattox D, Von Hoff D (1980) In vitro stem cell assay in head and neck squamous carcinoma. Am J Surg 140: 527-530
Mendelsohn M, Dethlefsen L (1968) Tumour growth and cellular kinetics. In: The proliferation and spread of neoplastic cells. Williams and Wilkins, Baltimore, pp 197-212
Meyskens F, Salmon S (1979) Inhibition of human melanoma colony formation by retinoids. Cancer Res 40: 4055-4057
Mihich E, Lawrence D, Lawrence D, Eckhardt S (1979) UICC workshop in human tumour sampling for biochemical pharmacological studies of target determinants of drug action. UICC Technical Report Series 43
Morgan G, Williams CJ, Smallwood J, Taylor I, Whitehouse J (1983) Colony-forming cells from primary tumours. Influence of dissociation method on colony growth in vitro. Proc AACR 24: 4 (abstr)
Omura G, Morrow C, Blessing J (1983) A randomised comparison of melphalan versus melphalan plus hexamethylmelamine versus adriamycin plus cyclophosphamide in ovarian carcinoma. Cancer 51: 783-789
Pollard E, Tio F, Myers J et al. (1981) Utilization of a human tumour cloning system to monitor for marrow involvement in small cell carcinoma of the lungs. Cancer Res 41: 1015-1020
Salmon S, Hamburger A, Soehnlen B, Durie B, Alberts D, Moon T (1978) Quantitation of differential sensitivity of human tumour stem cells to anti-cancer drugs. N Engl J Med 298: 1321-1327
Salmon S, Meyskens F, Alberts D, Soehnlen B, Young L (1981) New drugs in ovarian cancer and malignant melanoma: in vitro phase II screening with the human tumour stem cell assay. Cancer Treat Rep 65: 1-12
Salmon S, Von Hoff D, Williams CJ (1982) In vitro evaluation of anti-cancer drugs with the human tumour stem cell assay: In: C Williams, J Whitehouse (eds) Recent advances in clinical oncology. Churchill-Livingstone, Edinburgh
Sandbach J, Von Hoff D, Clark G, Cruz A, O'Brien M (1982) Direct cloning of human breast cancer in soft agar culture. Cancer 50: 1315-1321
Selby P, Steel G (1982) Use of the agar diffusion chamber for the exposure of human tumour cells to drugs. Cancer Res 42: 758-762
Selby P, Buick R, Tannock I (1983) A critical appraisal of the human tumour stem-cell assay. N Engl J Med 308: 129-134
Slocum H, Pavelic Z, Kantar P, Novak N, Rustum Y (1981) The soft agar clonogenicity and characterization of cells obtained from solid human tumours by mechanical and enzymatic methods. Cancer Chemother Pharmacol 6: 265-271

Smallwood J, Morgan G, Cooper A, Kirkham N, Williams C, Whitehouse J, Taylor I (1984) Correlations between clonogenicity and prognostic factors in human breast cancer. Br J Surg 71: 109-111
Steel G (1977) Growth kinetics of tumours: cell population kinetics in relation to the growth and treatment of cancer. Clarendon Press, Oxford
Sutherland C, Mather F, Carter R, Cerise E, Krementz E (1983) Breast cancer as analyzed by the human tumour stem cell assay. Surgery 94: 370-375
Tobias J, Griffiths C (1976) Management of ovarian carcinoma: Current concepts and future prospects. N Engl J Med 294: 818-823, 877-882
Uttendal M, Hubers H, McVie J, Pinedo H (1983) Human tumour clonogenicity in agar is improved by cell-free ascites. Br J Cancer 48: 55-59
Vogl S, Pagano M, Kaplan B (1983) Cisplatin based combination therapy for advanced ovarian cancer: High overall response rate with curative potential only in women with small tumour burdens. Cancer 51: 2024-2038
Von Hoff D (1983) Send this patient's tumour for culture and sensitivity. N Engl J Med 308: 154-155
Von Hoff D, Bradley E (1979) Use of human tumour stem cell assay to screen for phase II activity of new antineoplastic drugs. Eleventh International Congress of Chemotherapy, p 920
Von Hoff D, Rozencweig M, Muggia F (1979) Evaluation of cytotoxic drugs. Cancer Treat Rep 6: 1-8
Von Hoff D, Sandbach J, Osborne C, Metelmann C, Clark G, O'Brien M (1981 a) Potential and problems with growth of breast cancer in a human tumour cloning system. Breast Cancer Res Treat 1: 141-148
Von Hoff D, Cowan J, Harris G, Reisdorf G (1981 b) Human tumour cloning: Feasibility and clinical correlations. Cancer Chemother Pharmacol 6: 265-271
Von Hoff D, Capser J, Bradley E, Sandback J, Jones D, Makuch R (1981 c) Association between human colony-forming assay results and response of an individual patient's tumour to chemotherapy. Am J Med 70: 1027-1037
Von Hoff D, Page C, Harris G, Clark G, Cowan J, Coltman C (1982) Prospective clinical trial of a human tumour cloning system. Proc AACR 22: 154
Wasserman J, Comis R, Goldsmith M et al. (1975) Tabular analysis of the clinical course of chemotherapy of solid tumours. Cancer Chemother Rep, part 3, 6: 399-419
Welander C, Alberts D (1985) Clonogenic assay studies of tumour cells from gynecologic malignancies. In: C Williams, J Whitehouse (eds) Cancer investigation and management: female reproductive system. Wiley, Chichester
Welander C, Homesley H, Jobson V (1983) In vitro chemotherapy testing of gynecologic tumours: Basis for planning therapy. Am J Obstet Gynecol 147: 188-195
Williams C, Mead G, Arnold A (1982) Chemotherapy of advanced ovarian carcinoma: Initial experience using a platinum-based combination. Cancer 49: 1778-1783
Williams C, Mead G, Green J (1983 a) A randomised study of cisplatin, adriamycin and cyclophosphamide (PACe) versus chlorambucil (CB) in stage III and IV ovarian carcinoma. Proc ASCO 2: C-611 (Abstr)
Williams C, Smallwood J, Morgan G, Taylor I, Whitehouse J (1983 b) Influence of growth characteristics and hormone receptor status on clonogenicity of human breast cancer. Proc AACR 24: 675 (Abstr)

Chemotherapy in a Single Centre

E. Wiltshaw*

The Gynaecological Cancer Unit, Royal Marsden Hospital, London, United Kingdom

Interest in the treatment of ovarian cancer by chemotherapy in my Department goes back to the late 1950s when single, oral alkylating agents came into clinical practice. At that time, we were presented with only the very advanced stage III cases and some of the patients with stage IV disease, while the majority of our patients had recurrent disease following radiotherapy. However, in 1965 we were able to publish a series of 72 patients treated with chlorambucil (Wiltshaw 1965 a, b). This study showed that in the very advanced cases ascites was controlled better by chlorambucil than by radioactive colloidal gold, and that clinical responses were seen in patients given low-dose oral chemotherapy (Table 1). These were exciting results, particularly since epithelial ovarian tumours were the first adenocarcinomas in which it was shown consistently that approximately 26% clinical complete regressions could be produced by drugs (Table 2). Unfortunately, these responses were not accompanied by long-term survival and cure, and most of our 36 patients treated

Table 1. Control of ovarian ascites by radioactive gold or chlorambucil

Therapy	Free of ascites for >3 months (%)	Survival of >6 months after developing ascites (%)	Total no. cases
^{198}Au	13	21	58
Chlorambucil	31	41	23

Table 2. Response to chlorambucil in 62 ovarian cancer patients with measurable disease

	Complete regression	Partial or minimal regression
Type of response	16 (26%)	22 (35%)
Length of remission	Range 3-30 months (median 9 months)	

* Many people have been involved in these trials over the years, and I would like to acknowledge my gratitude to our collaborating surgeons and radiotherapists; also to Bristol Myers for a free supply of JM8 and cisplatin in the early days. Some of the studies were also supported more actively by both Bristol Myers and Johnson Mathey. I would also like to thank the many doctors and nurses on my team for their unfailing help and enthusiasm. Lastly, the patients are the true heroines, since they accepted all that we asked of them despite the eventual failure seen in most cases

Ovarian Cancer, Ed. by N. M. Bleehen

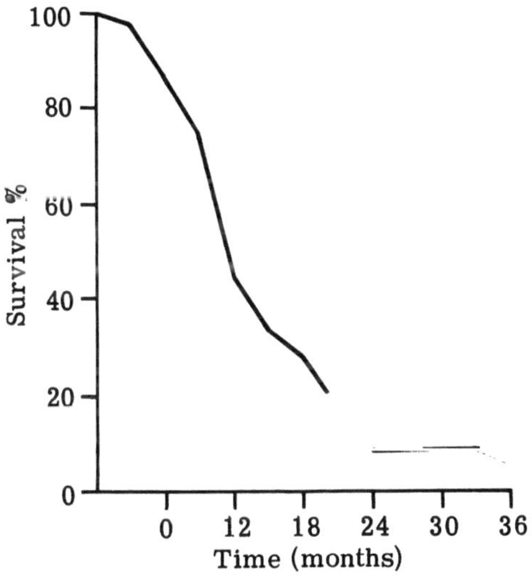

Fig. 1. Survival of 36 patients with stage III and IV ovarian cancer treated by chlorambucil alone post-operatively

post-operatively for stage III and IV disease had died within 3 years of chemotherapy (Fig. 1).

Later studies with melphalan, 5-fluorouracil, cyclophosphamide and busulphan confirmed that results would be similar with all these agents, and these results were obtained worldwide. At that time we also learned that once the first chemotherapeutic agent had failed, either because of initial resistance or because of relapse, further therapy with other agents was only very rarely of benefit.

Thus it was of special interest to be presented with a new agent of unknown potential, namely cisplatin, to try in our failed cases. This drug was introduced to us, with some enthusiasm, by the late Sir Alexander Haddow, on the basis that it had antitumour properties and yet was a completely different agent to those that preceded it. By this time our unit had considerable experience in the management of ovarian cancer, and because of this we recognised early the unusual property of cisplatin in producing second remissions in ovarian cancer after failure of single or combination chemotherapy with other agents. We were also lucky to have introduced, at an early stage in our studies, the use of intravenous hydration to protect the kidneys and to reduce the problems of severe vomiting. In 1974 we reported our preliminary results which showed a response rate of 27% in a series of 32 cases of previously treated patients (Wiltshaw and Kroner 1976). When this study was enlarged to 52 patients, the overall response rate was the same but the complete remission rate was shown to be 6% (Table 3).

Later use of higher doses of cisplatin in previously treated patients suggested that responses could be increased from 27% to 50% and complete remissions from 6% to 25%. These remissions lasted from 5 to 31 months (median 10 months) and were of good quality once the therapy was completed (Barker and Wiltshaw 1981 a).

Following our very early phase II study with cisplatin at 25–50 mg/m^2 in 1974 we started a randomised phase III study, the details of which are given in Table 4. We started by comparing cisplatin plus chlorambucil (regimen B) with chlorambucil alone (regimen A). After 34 patients had been entered there were only partial responses in the chlorambucil only arm, and the unit felt that this arm should be abandoned in favour of a combination of chlorambucil, cisplatin and doxorubucin (regimen C). Response rates and

Table 3. Response of advanced ovarian cancer to cisplatin

Cisplatin regimen	Responses (%)[a]		No. cases
	CR	PR	
30 mg/m^2 q 21 days	6	20	52
100 mg/m^2 q 28 days	25	29	31

[a] CR, complete regression; PR, partial regression

Table 4. Treatment regimens of a phase III chemotherapy study for late ovarian cancer

A Chlorambucil 0.2 mg/kg/per day × 14 days q 28 for 2 years

B Chlorambucil 0.15 mg/kg/per day × 7 days q 28 for 1 year
followed by 0.2 mg/kg/per day × 14 days q 28 for a further year
Cisplatin 20 mg/m^2 intravenously q 28 days for 12 courses

C Chlorambucil as in B
Cisplatin as in B
Doxorubicin 50 mg/m^2 intravenously with cisplatin q 28 days for 9 courses

D Cisplatin 100 mg/m^2 intravenously q 28 days for 10 courses

survival were reported in 1981 for regimens B and C (Barker and Wiltshaw 1981 b). There were 52% responders in regimen B with 28% complete remissions, and the addition of doxorubicin did not improve these figures (54% and 28% respectively). Thus it was concluded that doxorubicin added nothing to the therapeutic benefit of a combination of cisplatin and chlorambucil. Survival in this study confirmed this view and showed that survival was greatest for complete responders (65% at 3 years) while non-responders were all dead within 14 months.

The next logical step was to compare cisplatin at the higher, perhaps more effective, dose of 100 mg/m^2 with the older regimen B combination. Results of this study have not yet been published, but the response rates and survivals of patients randomised to regimen B are similar to our previous experience. Single-agent high-dose cisplatin (regimen D) again shows a 50% response rate and 27% complete remission rate, but there is an apparent survival benefit for single-agent cisplatin for stage III patients only.

During this trial The Institute of Cancer Research, in collaboration with the pharmaceutical industry, was investigating the possibility of using other platinum analogues for anti-tumour activity. Professor Harrap and Dr H. Calvert at The Institute of Cancer Research chose the analogue cis-diammine-I, I-cyclobutane dicarboxylate platinum II (JM8) for clinical testing. The reasons for the choice were that whilst the drug retained anti-tumour effects in animals, its most striking feature was the reduction in nephrotoxicity. In collaboration with Dr Calvert we embarked on a phase I and phase II study of this compound in man. To our surprise and delight we found that patients previously treated with cisplatin did sometimes have good further remissions following JM8. Data on 38 patients with ovarian cancer were published in 1982 (Calvert et al. 1982) and later more details were given on 36 patients (Evans et al. 1983). In patients treated previously with multiple other drugs, the response rate was 25%. Also, and most importantly, there was a suggestion that tumours were not always cross-resistant between JM8 and cisplatin. It was of

Table 5. Effect of JM8 on 33 patients previously treated with cisplatin

	No. of cases	Total evaluated
Response[a]	CR 2	
	PR 5	33
Bone marrow toxicity		
Total leucocyte count $< 1 \times 10^{a}/l$	6	33
Platelets $< 100 \times 10^{a}/l$	20	33
Requiring blood transfusion	14	33
Renal toxicity		
Reduction in EDTA clearance of $> 20\%$	3	22
Neurological toxicity		
Neuropathy	2	26[b]
Ototoxicity	0	33

[a] CR, complete remission; PR, partial remission
[b] Neuropathy only occurred in patients who had experienced neuropathy in previous cisplatin therapy

special value to patients that renal toxicity and neurological toxicity were almost non-existent (Table 5).
At the present time the unit is involved in a phase III trial of JM8 versus cisplatin in stage III and IV disease. Preliminary results suggest that the anti-tumour efficacy, in the short term, is similar for both compounds (Wiltshaw et al. 1983). Over one hundred patients have been entered in the trial to date, and there is no survival advantage with the new drug but toxicity and side-effects have been substantially reduced. However, JM8 has much greater myelosuppressing effects than cisplatin, and its dose must be related to renal function as well as to bone marrow reserve.

In summary, the ovarian unit at the Royal Marsden Hospital has studied, in some depth, the value of alkylating agents and platinum compounds in late-stage ovarian adenocarcinoma over a 20-year period. We believe that the survival of stage III patients has been improved, but have yet to show that the overall survival in ovarian cancer of all stages has benefited from modern management.

References

Barker GH, Wiltshaw E (1981 a) Use of high dose *cis*-dichlorodiammine platinum (II) (NSC-II9875) following failure on previous chemotherapy for advanced carcinoma of the ovary. Br J Obstet Gynaecol 88: 1192

Barker GH, Wiltshaw E (1981 b) Randomised trial comparing low-dose cisplatin and chlorambucil with low-dose cisplatin, chlorambucil and doxorubicin in advanced ovarian carcinoma. Lancet I: 747

Calvert AH, Harland SJ, Newell DR, Siddik ZH et al. (1982) Early clinical studies with *cis*-diammine-I,I-cyclobutane dicarboxylate platinum II. Cancer Chemother Pharmacol 9: 140

Evans B, Raju KS, Calvert AH, Harland SJ, Wiltshaw E (1983) Phase II study of JM8, a new platinum analog, in advanced ovarian carcinoma. Cancer Treat Rep 67: 997

Wiltshaw E (1965 a) Chlorambucil in the treatment of primary adenocarcinoma of the ovary. J Obstet Gynaecol Br Cwlth 72: 586
Wiltshaw E (1965 b) A retrospective comparison of chlorambucil and radiotherapy in the treatment of ovarian adenocarcinoma. J Obstet Gynaecol Br Cwlth 72: 595
Wiltshaw E, Kroner T (1976) Phase II study of *cis*-dichlorodiammine platinum II (NSC-119875) in advanced adenocarcinoma of the ovary. Cancer Treat Rep 60: 55
Wiltshaw E, Evans BD, Baker JW, Calvert AH, Jones AC (1983) JM8, successor to cisplatin in advanced ovarian carcinoma. Lancet I: 587 (letter)

Chemotherapy in Multicentre Studies

D. Guthrie*

Regional Radiotherapy Centre, Newcastle General Hospital, Newcastle upon Tyne, United Kingdom

It has long been recognized that patients with advanced epithelial carcinoma of the ovary have a very poor prognosis, with very few surviving to 5 years (Aure et al. 1971). The possibility of improving survival with modern chemotherapy has always seemed tenable in view of the high remission rates that can be obtained with such drugs, but to date such an improvement has not been conclusively demonstrated. In this chapter the evolution of such chemotherapy will be traced, leading ultimately to a detailed analysis of certain large-scale multicentre studies. It will be seen that studies are frequently based on the assumption that the treatment which produces the greatest remission rate is the one that is best for the patient, but this may not necessarily be true: an evaluation based on survival and quality of life is of far greater potential benefit to the patient.

Single-Agent Therapy

Table 1 is taken from the excellent two-part article by Tobias and Griffiths (1976) and lists the drugs most commonly used in treating ovarian cancer. The combined partial and complete remission rates shown must be regarded as approximate, and in this respect platinum compounds would now have a higher placing. Table 2 shows the results that can be obtained with some of these drugs. It will be seen immediately that there is a wide variation in remission rate but surprisingly little variation in the duration of remission or survival. The variation in remission rate is due in part to variation in the method of assessment, but also to variation in dose, there being reasonable evidence to suggest that the response to single-agent alkylating agents is dose dependent; but dose, of course, is limited by toxicity. Little toxicity, was experienced by the patients receiving melphalan 0.2 mg/kg daily for 5 days in the study reported by Piver et al. (1978) or in the study of Mangioni et al. (1976), where patients received cyclophosphamide 50 mg twice daily, but in both these studies response rates were relatively poor. In contrast, Geisler et al. (1976) succeeded in producing a very high combined partial and complete remission rate of 89% by administering up to 4 g cyclophosphamide IV every 4 weeks. Such treatment produced an 81% overall survival at 12 months but at the expense of a marked increase in toxicity: all patients had nausea and vomiting for 24–36 h after treatment and even though all of

* I wish to thank Alain Maskens, Jan Vermorken, Marie van der Burg, Nicole Rotmensz and Otilia Dalesio for permission to publish the results of the EORTC Gynaecological Cancer Group Study. The levamisole trial was supported by the North of England Council of the Cancer Campaign

Ovarian Cancer, Ed. by N. M. Bleehen

Table 1. Remission rates for single agent cytotoxic therapy in ovarian cancer

Alkylating agents	50%
Hexamethylmelamine	40%
Adriamycin	35%
Methotrexate	30%
Platinum compounds	25%
5-Fluorouracil	20%
Vinblastine	20%

Table 2. Cytotoxic therapy in carcinoma of the ovary

Number of patients	Complete remission rate	Partial remission rate	Drugs used	Source
89	13% (19S)	11% (11S)	Melphalan	Piver et al. (1978)
72	15% (17R)	26% (8R)	Cyclo	Mangioni et al. (1976)
26	77% (18R)	12% (8R)	Cyclo	Geisler et al. (1976)
54	46% (15R)	30% (7R)	Cyclo + Depostat	Guthrie (1978)
25	20% (11R)	36% (7R)	VCN + ACT D + MTX + Cyclo	Kessinger et al. (1976)
29	31% (18R)	38% (−)	Cyclo + 5FU	Izbicki et al. (1977)
14	36% (10R)	43% (5 + R)	ADR + Cyclo	Lloyd et al. (1976)
41	49% (9R)	34% (7R)	ADR + Cyclo	Parker et al. (1980)

Median duration of remission (R) or survival (S) is given in parentheses in months
Key: Cyclo, cyclophosphamide; VCN, vincristine; ACT D, actinomycin D; MTX, methotrexate; 5FU, 5-fluorouracil; ADR, Adriamycin (doxorubicin)

them consumed at least 3 litres of fluid per day, 19% developed a severe haemorrhagic cystitis. My own work with cyclophosphamide and Depostat (gestronol hexanoate) did not give quite such a high remission rate, but toxicity was considerably less (Guthrie 1979). The Depostat was included because some patients with ovarian cancer will respond to a progestogen alone and progestogens have the added advantage of inducing a feeling of well-being in patients.

Multiple-Agent Treatment

In the area of multiple-agent treatment Kessinger et al. (1976) added vincristine, actinomycin D and methotrexate to cyclophosphamide with no evidence of increased efficacy, although as expected the combination was toxic. In contrast, the addition of 5-fluorouracil to cyclophosphamide, as reported by Izbicki et al. (1977), was reasonably effective, but at the expense of toxicity. Treatment lasted 4 days and produced stomatitis, nausea, vomiting and thrombophlebitis. The papers by Lloyd et al. (1976) and Parker et al. (1980) both showed that high remission rates with only moderate toxicity could be obtained with combinations of Adriamycin (doxorubicin) and cyclophosphamide, but unfortunately such remissions were of relatively short duration.

Comparative Trials of Single-Agent and Combination Chemotherapy

Having demonstrated that cytotoxic treatment could be effective many workers naturally progressed to phase III studies, usually in an effort to determine whether multiple-agent therapy was better than single-agent treatment. Many such studies are listed in Table 3. A common feature of all the studies listed in Table 3 is that although they differ in remission rate, none of them shows any evidence of improvement in survival.

The large Canadian national trial reported by Miller et al. (1980) differs from the others in that a comparison was made between giving all three drugs simultaneously and giving the same drugs sequentially, using each drug until progression before changing to the next. The median survival figures in Table 3 have been derived from survival curves in these authors' paper, which show no difference in survival between the two groups. Remission rates were similar, but surprisingly, the sequential regimen was more toxic than the combination regimen.

The four-arm study of the Gynecologic Oncology Group reported by Park et al. (1980) is shown in part in Table 3; only those patients who did not have prior radiotherapy are referred to. Again remission rates are similar, and although the survival figures derived from the paper appear to differ there is virtually no difference between the various survival curves for the different arms. Toxicity for the different regimens was similar, except that leucopenia was greater with the second and fourth regimens.

The studies reported by Turbow et al. (1980), Bolis et al. (1980), and Schwartz et al. (1981) were similar in that each had a combination of Adriamycin and cyclophosphamide

Table 3. Comparative studies in advanced ovarian cancer in which no significant differences in survival were found

Treatment	n	CR%	PR%	Median survival (months)	Source
L-PAM+5FU+MTX	119	24	16	14	Miller et al.
L-PAM→5FU→MTX	121	25	23	10	1980
L-PAM	61	20	10	9	Park et al.
L-PAM+5FU	48	17	8	13	1980
L-PAM+5FU+ACT D	48	17	15	13	
CYCLO+5FU+ACT D	21	10	24	8	
L-PAM	23	13	17	14	Turbow et al.
ADR+CYCLO	24	58	13	14	1980
CYCLO	33	12	30	13	Bolis et al.
ADR+CYCLO	33	18	33	14	1980
HMM+CYCLO	20	30	20	14	Schwartz et al.
ADR+CYCLO	17	35	24	17	1981
CYCLO	131	–22–			Medical Research
CYCLO+HMM+MTX	130	–33–			Council 1981
L-PAM	64	20	17	12	Omura et al.
L-PAM+HMM	97	28	24	14	1983
ADR+CYCLO	72	32	17	14	

Key: L-PAM, melphalan; 5FU, 5-fluorouracil; MTX, methotrexate; ACT D, actinomycin D; CYCLO, cyclophosphamide; ADR, Adriamycin (doxorubicin); HMM, hexamethylmelamine

Table 4. Toxicity recorded in the Medical Research Council trial in advanced ovarian cancer (1981)

	CYCLO ($n=131$)	CYCLO + HMM + MTX ($n=130$)
Protocol deviation	27%	65%
Protocol substantially modified or abandoned	14%	44%
Alopecia	5%	28%

Key: CYCLO, cyclophosphamide; HMM, hexamethylmelamine; MTX, methotrexate
Protocol deviation, substantial modification or abandonment all relate to such action being taken as a result of toxicity

for one of the two regimens being compared. It will be seen that in each of these studies the Adriamycin-cyclophosphamide had a higher remission rate than the other arm, but yet again, this increase in remission rate did not affect survival, there being no difference in survival between the two arms in any of these trials. Unfortunately the increase in remission was obtained at the expense of increased toxicity, the Adriamycin-cyclophosphamide combination being much more toxic than the other regimen in each of these studies.

Similar findings hold true for the large multicentre study of the Medical Research Council in the United Kingdom (Medical Research Council's Working Party on Ovarian Cancer 1981). In this study response was defined as a reduction of more than 50% in the total tumour mass at 6 months from the start of treatment. Oral cyclophosphamide 100 mg daily was compared with a three-drug regimen, namely cyclophosphamide 100 mg PO twice daily on days 1-14 inclusive, together with hexamethylmelamine 100 mg twice daily on days 1-14 inclusive and methotrexate 50 mg PO on days 1 and 80. This combination of drugs was repeated on a cyclical basis every 4 weeks.

It can be seen from Table 3 that the response rate at 6 months was much greater for the triple-chemotherapy arm than for the single-agent arm, but as shown in Table 4, this was achieved at the expense of increased toxicity.

Even for the simple side effect of alopecia, it can be seen that there was a much greater chance of this occurring with the triple-chemotherapy arm that with cyclophosphamide alone. A quantitative assessment of toxicity has also been made, toxicity being recorded when it was sufficient to cause protocol deviation or to necessitate substantial modification or even abandonment of the protocol. When the results are examined with this in mind it can be seen that the differences between the two arms of the study were very marked, toxicity always being greater in the triple-agent arm.

Although the toxicity was obviously greater in patients treated with the triple-agent combination it may be reasonable to accept this if the increase in remission rate is translated into an increase in the length of survival. Figure 1 shows the overall survival curves for the two arms of the trial, and yet again there is not even an intermediate gap between the two curves.

In the later study of the Gynecologic Oncology Group (Omura et al. 1983) again a simple alkylating agent was used as the reference regimen, and again, another arm received a combination containing hexamethylmelamine: in the third arm the Adriamycin-cyclophosphamide combination is again seen. Patients eligible for this study were those with histologically proven ovarian carcinoma of epithelial origin, either FIGO stage IV or recurrent, or with stage III disease in which residual lesions after surgery were equal to or greater than 3 cm in the largest diameter. Patients with a Karnofsky performance status of less than 40% were not admitted to this trial. Patients were stratified by measurable versus

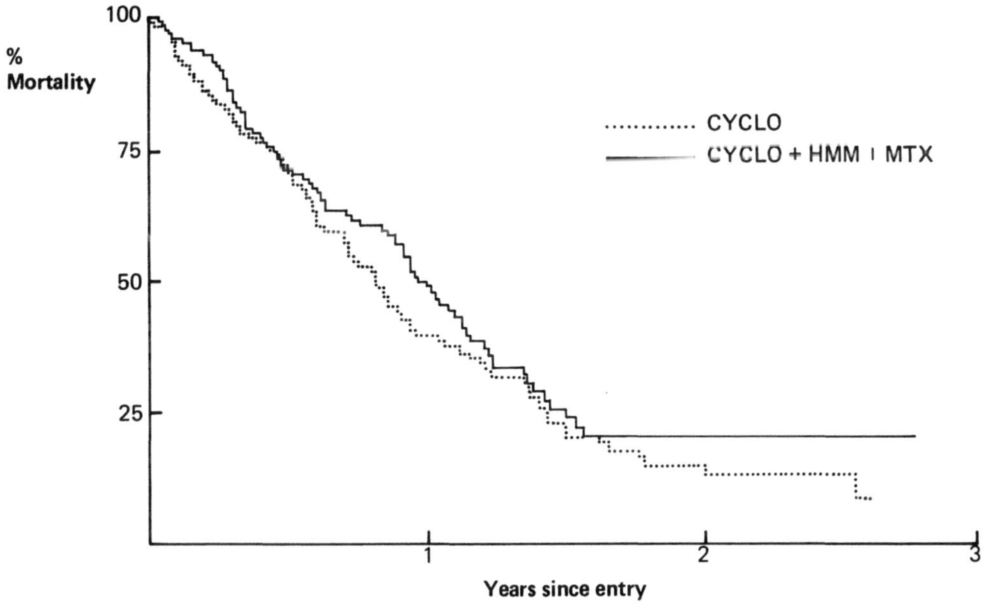

Fig. 1. Medical Research Council Advanced Ovarian Cancer Study (1981). Survival curves of overall mortality by allocated treatment. The continuous line represents the survival experience of 130 patients treated with a combination of cyclophosphamide, hexamethylmelamine and methotrexate. The dotted line represents the survival experience of 131 patients treated with cyclophosphamide alone

non-measurable disease, and by prior radiotherapy or no prior radiotherapy, and each was then randomly assigned to one of three treatment groups, these being either melphalan 7 mg/m^2 PO daily for 5 days or the same dose of melphalan together with hexamethylmelamine, the dose here being 150 mg/m^2 daily for 14 days: both treatment regimens were repeated on a 4-weekly basis. The third arm received Adriamycin 50 mg/m^2 together with cyclophosphamide 500 mg/m^2, both given IV once every 3 weeks. The Adriamycin was stopped after nine courses and the treatment continued with cyclophosphamide alone, the dose being increased by 25% with each successive course up to a maximum of 1100 mg/m^2. In all arms of the trial, treatment was stopped at 18 months. The results (Table 3) show that the combination of melphalan and hexamethylemelamine produces a higher complete remission rate than the melphalan alone, but the highest complete remission rate of all is that produced by the Adriamycin-cyclophosphamide combination. Although a total of 432 patients were entered in this study, the results refer to the 233 patients who had measurable disease subsequent to primary laparotomy. Table 5 shows that in virtually all situations the increase in remission rate has been bought at the expense of a marked increase in toxicity, the only exception being the incidence of thrombocytopenia in relation to the Adriamycin-cyclophosphamide arm. Again does the increase in remission with its associated toxicity produce a worthwhile increase in length of survival? Reference to Fig. 2 shows that it does not, there being no difference in the three survival curves. At this stage, it could be argued that the aforementioned trials are not fully relevant insofar as they do not include the use of cisplatin, which may be regarded as the drug of choice in the treatment of patients with advanced ovarian cancer. Many presume that use of this drug automatically leads to an increase in survival - but is this so?

Table 5. Toxicity recorded in the Gynecologic Oncology Group trial in advanced ovarian cancer (1983)

	Melphalan	Melphalan +HMM	ADR+CYCLO
WCC < $2.0 \times 10^9/1$	10%	23%	34%
Platelets < $50 \times 10^9/1$	12%	16%	2%
Vomiting	10%	36%	57%
Minimum numbers	89	137	104

Key: HMM, hexamethylmelamine; ADR, Adriamycin (doxorubicin); CYCLO, cyclophosphamide

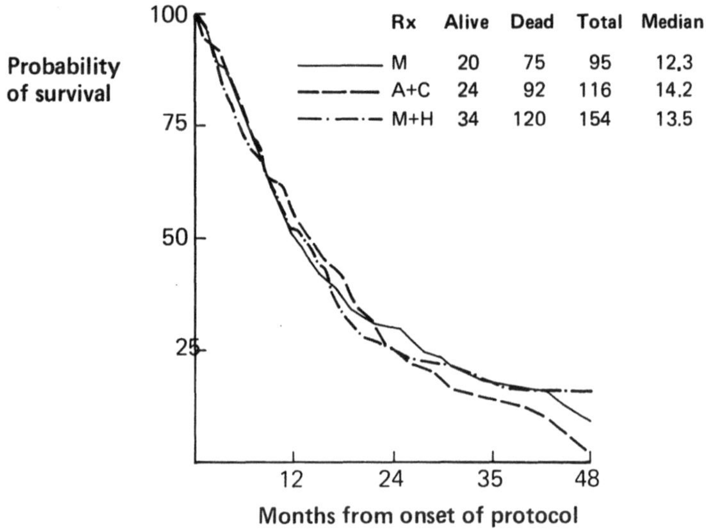

Fig. 2. Gynecologic Oncology Group Advanced Ovarian Cancer Study (1983). Survival by therapy for all evaluable patients. Drugs: melphalan (M); Adriamycin (doxorubicin) (A); cyclophosphamide (C); hexamethylmelamine (H)

Table 6 gives the results of comparative studies in advanced ovarian cancer in which one arm of each study received a regimen containing cisplatin. Again all studies have a common feature, in that although there are marked differences in remission rates none of the studies shows any evidence of improvement in survival. The study reported by Carmo-Pereira et al. (1982) differs from all the others in that it was the single-agent cyclophosphamide arm that had the higher remission rate, whereas in all the other studies the multiple-agent arm receiving combinations containing cisplatin had most remissions. Once more, the increase in remission rate was achieved at the expense of a marked increase of toxicity, the multiple-agent regimens containing cisplatin being much more toxic in all the studies. Such an increase in remission rate with its associated toxicity does not produce any improvement in survival in any of the studies. The results of the large EORTC Gynaecological Cancer Group Study (Maskens et al. 1983) may be used to illustrate this point in detail.

Patients with stage III or IV ovarian cancer of epithelial origin were randomized to receive Adriamycin 45 mg/m^2 together with cyclophosphamide 600 mg/m^2 IV every 4 weeks for 1 year, or the same two drugs in the same dosage, together with cisplatin

Table 6. Comparative studies in advanced ovarian cancer in which no significant differences in survival were found

Treatment	n	CR%	PR%	Median survival (Months)	Source
CYCLO	27	–66–		12	Carmo-Pereira et al. 1982
HMM+ADR+DDP	26	–38–		11	
ADR+CYCLO	101	20	26	No significant difference	Omura et al. 1982
ADR+CYCLO+DDP	91	44	27		
CHLORAMBUCIL	27	–26–		17	Williams et al. 1983
ADR+CYCLO+DDP	27	–72–			
CYCLO	35	21	33	14	Wagstaff et al. 1983
CYCLO+BLEO+DDP	41	23	50		
ADR+CYCLO	54	24	24		Maskens et al. 1983
ADR+CYCLO+DDP	55	38	18		

All studies have one arm treated with a combination including cisplatin
Key: CYCLO, cyclophosphamide; HMM, hexamethylmelamine; DDP, cisplatin; BLEO, bleomycin

Table 7. Toxicity recorded in the EORTC trial in advanced ovarian cancer (1983)

	ADR+CYCLO (n = 61)	ADR+CYCLO+DDP (n = 64)
Severe alopecia	55%	61%
Severe vomiting	26%	54%
Renal	4%	19%
Infection	7%	16%
Mucous	0%	14%
Bleeding	2%	12%
Neurological	4%	8%

Key: ADR, adriamycin (doxorubicin); CYCLO, cyclophosphamide; DDP, cisplatin

50 mg/m^2. At the end of 1 year a laparotomy was to be performed in responding or clinically disease-free patients. In all, 156 patients have been entered in this study, 109 of whom were evaluable for response. Table 6 shows that once again the multiple-agent regimen produced a higher complete response rate, but that again, this higher response rate had been bought at the expense of greater toxicity, as shown in Table 7. It can be seen from this table that for all the listed toxicities the cisplatin-containing arm is the more toxic of the two. Reference to Fig. 3 shows that the increase in remission with its associated toxicity does not produce a worthwhile increase in the length of survival. Figure 3 relates to the entire group of patients, but further analyses of survival curves have been made in subgroups comprising responders only, those patients with extended surgery, or those with limited surgery, and in all these subgroups again no difference has been found in the survival curves.

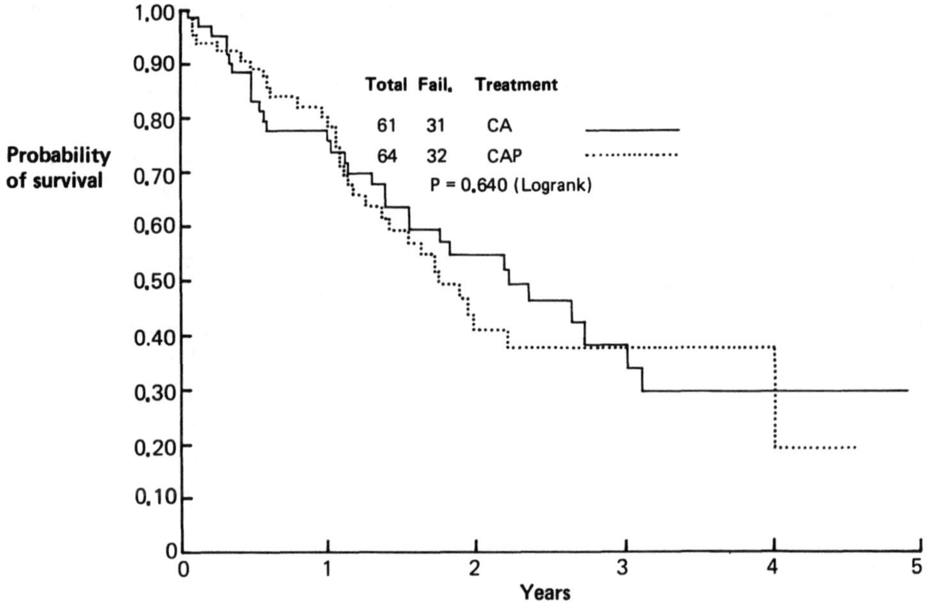

Number of patients at risk at the corresponding times

61	40	20	9	2	0	CA
64	44	15	4	2	0	CAP

Fig. 3. EORTC Gynaecological Cancer Group Advanced Ovarian Cancer Study (1983): Overall probability of survival by treatment group. The continuous line represents those patients treated with a combination of Adriamycin (doxorubicin) and cyclophosphamide (CA). The dotted line represents the survival probability of patients treated with Adriamycin (doxorubicin) plus cyclophosphamide plus cisplatin (CAP)

Questions to Be Asked in Analysing Clinical Trials

The results of the trials presented so far demonstrate that a very careful decision must be made as to the question a clinical trial in advanced ovarian cancer is designed to answer. It is my belief that we should put ourselves in the patient's situation. What the patient wants to know is "Will the treatment prolong my life?" and furthermore, "What will the quality of life be like during the course of my treatment?" It may be very gratifying for the doctor to see a tumour disappear when assessed by our present very crude methods, but as we have seen, such disappearance of tumour does little to help the patient as regards survival. It is essential that we remember at all times that we are treating patients who happen to have cancer and not cancers that happen to have patients attached.

Figure 4 illustrates one method by which we may be able to examine the results of clinical trials in future, whereby the effects of treatment are judged in terms of quality of life and survival. In Fig. 4 treatment B is seen to produce a 50% prolongation of survival, but compared with the results of treatment A the quality of life during this increased survival time is very poor. For example, the patient could be in hospital for many days every month receiving her treatment: such treatment may be accompanied by nausea and vomiting coupled with general malaise and the indignity of alopecia. However, the patient

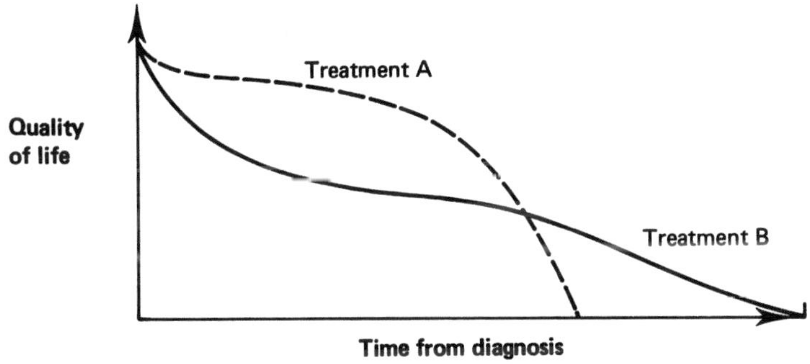

Fig. 4. Curves depicting quality of life by length of survival. Treatment B prolonged survival by 50% but is not regarded as beneficial to the patient as it involves a significant decrease in the quality of life when compared with treatment A

who is receiving treatment A may well be treated on an out-patient basis only, coming to hospital once a month for a full blood count but subjected to little inconvenience in any other way. It can be seen that when treatment A ceases to be effective the patient rapidly succumbs to her illness, as opposed to the lingering experienced by the patient receiving treatment B. From a mathematical point of view, treatment A can be compared with treatment B by measuring and comparing the areas under the two curves. In the example given, the area under the curve for treatment A is greater than that for treatment B. Treatment A is, therefore, superior when judged by this means. It is my firm belief that a method of analysis which combines length of survival with quality of life should be used in future trials, to enable clinicians to evaluate our treatments more carefully with regard to the requirements of patients.

Trials in Which Improvement in Survival is Claimed

Hexa CAF (Hexamethylmelamine + cyclophosphamide + methotrexate + 5-fluorouracil)

In 1978 Young et al. published work which claimed to show for the first time that an increase in survival could be obtained by using a multiple-agent regimen (Hexa CAF) as opposed to a single alkylating agent alone. Some of the results from that paper are shown in Table 8. A superficial inspection of these results suggests that the higher remission rate achieved with the four-drug regimen was effective in producing a marked improvement in the overall length of survival. However, the work was subsequently heavily criticised on the basis of statistical method and unequal distribution of histological grading by Barlow and Blumenson (1979) and Bush (1979).

Subsequent workers have examined the same four-drug combination in the hope of repeating the apparent success, and these results are summarized in the remainder of Table 8. In the paper by Neijt et al. (1980) the figure for the overall median survival is not given, but that for the patients who achieved partial remission is given as 8 months (range 3–25) and all the complete remission patients were alive and disease free at 7, 13, 22, 25, and 35 months at the time of reporting. The authors note that their results were not as good as those of Young et al. (1978), but thought that this could be due to their having fewer patients with lesions of less than 2 cm diameter after primary surgery.

Table 8. Studies of Hexa-CAF in advanced ovarian cancer

Treatment	n	CR%	PR%	Median survival (months)	Source
L-PAM	37	16	38	17	Young et al. 1978
HMM+CYCLO+MTX +5FU	40	33	43	29	
HMM+CYCLO+MTX +5FU	23	22	30	>8	Neijt et al. 1980
CYCLO	29	24	38	11	Carmo-Pereira et al. 1981
HMM+CYCLO+MTX +5FU	28	14	21	10	
L-PAM	38	13	-	No significant difference	Sturgeon et al. 1982
HMM+CYCLO+MTX +5FU	37	19	-		
ADR+CYCLO +DDP	40	30	-		

Key: L-PAM, melphalan; HMM, hexamethylmelamine; CYCLO, cyclophosphamide; MTX, methotrexate; 5FU, 5-fluorouracil; ADR, Adriamycin (doxorubicin); DDP, cisplatin

The study of Carmo-Pereira et al. (1981) differs from the others in that the cyclophosphamide arm had significantly more remissions that the multiple-agent arm. There was no difference in the survival curves, however, median survival in the combination arm being very much less than that found by Young et al. Median survival figures are not given in the study of Sturgeon et al. (1982). In this three-arm study remission rates were again higher with the multiple-agent regimens, the highest being that for the cisplatin-containing arm, but in spite of this no significant difference was recorded in survival at 3 years when the three arms were compared.

In the studies depicted in Table 8, the multiple-agent regimen was always found to be much more highly toxic than the single-agent regimens. Again, such toxicity cannot be justified because the initial hope of improved survival has not been confirmed by subsequent studies.

Other Trials in Which Improvement in Survival is Claimed

A number of other trials claim improvement in survival, but unfortunately, the use of differing methods of reporting results does not allow comparative tables to be produced. The short report by Mangioni et al. (1981) concerned a comparative study of a combination of Adriamycin and cyclosphophamide coupled with either cisplatin or hexamethylmelamine. In this study 102 patients with advanced ovarian cancer were randomized. The arm receiving cisplatin had complete and partial remission rates of 53% and 25%, respectively, and in the arm treated with the combination containing hexamethylmelamine complete and partial remission rates of 43% and 35%, respectively, were achieved. Although the combined partial and complete remission rates in the two arms were identical at 78%, the disease-free survival at 1 year was statistically better with the regimen containing cisplatin, at 46%; that with the regimen containing hexamethylmelamine was only 9%. Unfortunately, details concerning the comparability of the patients in the two groups are not given, and hence the true significance of this result cannot be assessed: it is possible that unequal distribution of prognostic factors could account for the difference, and furthermore, as survival curves are not given it cannot be said whether there was a significant difference in overall survival.

Equally encouraging results were reported by Tropé on behalf of the Swedish Cooperative Ovarian Cancer Study Group (1981). In this study, patients were randomized to receive either melphalan alone or a combination of melphalan and Adriamycin. Among the 72 patients receiving melphalan alone, 7 complete remissions and 22 partial remissions were recorded, with an overall survival of 10.7 months. In contrast, 21 complete remissions and 23 partial remissions were obtained among the 70 patients receiving the combinations, the overall survival being significantly longer at 16.8 months. In general, this moderate increase in survival was achieved with little increase in toxicity, the combination having more side effects in general although melphalan alone was more toxic to the bone marrow. Once more, details concerning the comparability of the two groups were not given, and according to Neijt (1983) the results were severely criticised and could not be confirmed by others.

By its title, "Diamminedichloroplatinum-based Combination Chemotherapy is Superior to Melphalan for Advanced Ovarian Cancer when age, 50 and Tumor Diameter>-2 cms", the report by Vogl et al. (1982) on behalf of the Eastern Cooperative Oncology Group suggested that combination therapy was better than single agent treatment. The details of the short report lead to a different overall conclusion, however. In this study 253 patients were randomized to receive either melphalan alone or a combination of cisplatin, Adriamycin, cyclophosphamide, and hexamethylmelamine. In patients aged less than 50 years melphalan produced a 76% response rate and the combination a 78% response rate. In patients aged 50 years or over the comparable figures were 29% and 60%. Survival curves were not given but the median *projected* survival was 19 months for the combination and 17 months for melphalan. The authors noted that they had as yet failed to demonstrate advantages for those aged less than 50 years or with small tumour burdens, or to show that the combination prolonged survival. This paper illustrates that sufficiently frequent analysis of data very soon reveals by chance a carefully defined subgroup where there are differences in outcome, but such differences are usually not real, being more of a statistical quirk which does not relate in practice to overall management of ovarian cancer patients in general.

It is possible to support this interpretation by looking at the paper from the same group but published 1 year later (Vogl et al. 1983). In this later study, the same four-drug combination was used in identical dosage in 38 patients, but on this occasion they concluded that the combination had a curative potential only in women with a tumour burden of less than or equal to 2 cm.

The title of the paper by Bruckner et al. (1981), "Improved Chemotherapy for Ovarian Cancer with *cis*-Diamminedichloroplatinum and Adriamycin", again suggests results that are not fully supported by the content of the paper. The paper describes a comparative study in which 5 patients receive thio-TEPA, 12 patients a combination of thio-TEPA and methotrexate and 18 patients in each of the two remaining groups received either cisplatin or Adriamycin and cisplatin. The title relates to a subset of patients with poorly differentiated tumours or tumours of unknown grade, there being 7, 13, and 9 such patients in the cisplatin, Adriamycin-cisplatin and thio-TEPA-methotrexate groups, respectively. Better survival is claimed for cisplatin-containing regimens than for the thio-TEPA-methotrexate regimen, with a quoted *P* value of 0.01. Unfortunately, the groups were not strictly comparable, there being fewer patients with residual disease of 2 cm or less in the thio-TEPA-methotrexate group than the cisplatin-containing groups, and furthermore the performance status and age distribution favoured the cisplatin-containing groups. Hence, to claim the improvement suggested in the title of the article with such small numbers and bias in known prognostic variables could be regarded as a triumph of statistics over common sense.

The final sentence of the summary of the study by Decker et al. (1982) states: "The study demonstrates a striking superiority of combination chemotherapy over single-agent chemotherapy in patients with advanced ovarian cancer." In this study a comparison was made between patients treated with cyclophosphamide alone and those treated with a combination of cyclophosphamide and cisplatin. Of the 21 patients entered in each arm 13 were still alive in the combination group at 2 years, whereas only 4 patients were still alive in the cyclophosphamide group. This difference in survival is not significant according to a log-rank test, but is significant when other tests of significance are used.

Unfortunately, the two groups in this study were not strictly comparable, the most important difference being that in tumour bulk. In this respect twice as many patients in the cyclophosphamide arm had residual tumour nodules of 5 cm diameter as in the combination group. In addition to this, the cyclophosphamide arm contained more patients with poorly differentiated tumours than the combination arm. It is therefore unwise to base the subsequent management of ovarian cancer on the results reported in this small series, particularly in view of the differences noted in known prognostic factors between the two groups: a larger study with a more even distribution of prognostic variables should be undertaken to evaluate the suggested advantage of the combination chemotherapy, and until this has been done such absolute statements as that given in their summary should not be made.

Trials Involving Immunotherapy

There is little doubt that host defence mechanisms play a major role in ovarian cancer (Hudson 1980), but whether these can be adequately used to the advantage of the patient has been the subject of much research and subsequent debate.

Barlow et al. (1980) published the results of a study in which patients received either a combination of methotrexate and cyclophosphamide or a combination of 5-fluorouracil and cyclophosphamide. No difference was found between the two groups with regard to the median duration of response or survival: furthermore, 10 patients in each group also received *C. parvum* immunotherapy and this also was found not have any effect upon survival.

In contrast, Wilbur et al. (1983) used a different type of immunotherapeutic agent, namely BCG, in a study in which patients were randomized to receive either cyclophosphamide or cyclophosphamide plus cisplatin and then within each chemotherapy arm were further randomized to receive BCG or not. The median survival in the cyclophosphamide arm was 18 months and that for the cyclophosphamide plus cisplatin arm only 14 months, but the difference was not significant. However, a significant difference in survival was found between the patients who had BCG and those who did not. The median survival in these groups was 23 and 13 months, respectively. With only 24 patients admitted to this study at the time of the preliminary report, the authors' conclusion was understandably guarded: "This small study demonstrates no clear advantage for the addition of cisplatin to cyclophosphamide as initial chemotherapy for ovarian carcinoma but raises a question about a possible benefit of BCG."

An earlier much larger study by the Southwest Oncology Group (Alberts et al. 1979) showed a clear benefit in terms of survival for patients treated with BCG, and it is worth examining this trial in detail.

Southwest Oncology Group Study in Advanced Ovarian Cancer

Patients with epithelial carcinoma of the ovary, either stage III or IV disease or patients with recurrent disease subsequent to surgery or radiation were admitted to this study. All patients were treated with Adriamycin 40 mg/m^2 IV on day 1, followed by cyclophosphamide PO 200 mg/m^2 on days 3-6 inclusive, this treatment being repeated on a 3- to 4-weekly cycle basis. Patients were randomized to receive either no additional treatment or BCG scarification at alternating upper and lower extremity sites on days 8 and 15. After 12 cycles of treatment all patients thought to be in complete remission or partial remission with potentially resectable disease were subjected to a second-look laparotomy. After 1 year, all patients in complete or partial remission were treated by means of cyclophosphamide PO alone at a dose of 200 mg/m^2 daily for 5 days every 4 weeks for a further year. BCG scarification was continued on day 15 only when patients developed erythema and oedema beyond the margin of scarification and/or lymphadenopathy.

The results of this study are shown in Table 9. Of the 154 patients entered, 118 were evaluable for response. The results show that the addition of BCG scarification produced a statistically significant ($P = 0.05$) increase in response rate. The low complete response rate in both arms of the trial is a reflection of the extensive second-look laparotomy used as a means of formally assessing remission in patients at 1 year.

Table 10 shows that this increase in remission rate was achieved without any increase in conventional toxicity. BCG scarification itself produced little increase in toxicity and

Table 9. Responses recorded in the Southwest Oncology Group trial in advanced ovarian cancer (1979)

Number	Complete response (%)	Partial response (%)	Drugs used
57	12	40	ADR + CYCLO + BCG
61	2	34	ADR + CYCLO

Key: ADR, Adriamycin (doxorubicin); CYCLO, cyclophosphamide; BCG, *Bacillus Calmette-Guérin*

Table 10. Toxicity recorded in the Southwest Oncology Group trial in advanced ovarian cancer (1979)

	ADR + CYCLO + BCG	ADR + CYCLO
WCC $< 2.0 \times 10^9/1$	44%	41%
Platelets $< 75 \times 10^9/1$	11%	10%

Key: ADR, Adriamycin (doxorubicin); CYCLO, cyclophosphamide; BCG, *Bacillus Calmette-Guérin*

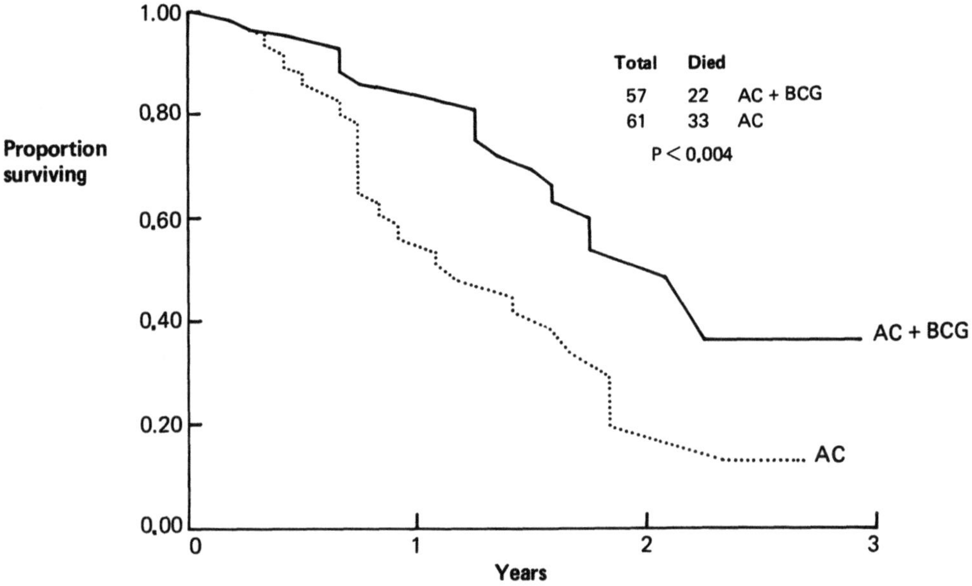

Fig. 5. Southwest Oncology Group Advanced Ovarian Cancer Study (1979): Actuarial survival from start of chemotherapy for 118 evaluable patients with stage III and IV tumours with measurable residual disease. The continuous line represents patients receiving Adriamycin (doxorubicin) plus cyclophosphamide together with BCG scarification (AC+BCG); the dotted line represents those patients who received Adriamycin (doxorubicin) plus cyclophosphamide alone (AC). Statistical analysis by Wilcoxon test

no patient experienced serious toxic effects, although 10 of the 57 evaluable patients who received BCG did experience some systemic side effects. Two patients developed erythema multiforme-type skin reactions, which resolved with steroid therapy but caused discontinuation of the BCG.

Figure 5 shows that for the first time there was a very marked difference in the survival curves when comparing the two groups. The median survival for the group which did not receive BCG scarification was only thirteen months whereas the BCG group had a median survival of almost 24 months. This difference is statistically significant ($P < 0.004$).

There is one other trial which shows improvement in survival in ovarian cancer patients treated with immunotherapy, the immunotherapeutic agent in this study being levamisole. The results of this study have not yet been published, but certain details are given below.

Levamisole Trial in Advanced Ovarian Cancer

This trial has been in progess on a multicentre basis in the North of England for the past 7 years. All patients admitted to this trial had advanced ovarian cancer of epithelial origin and all had residual disease after primary surgery. Patients were stratified by the extent of surgery, being divided simply into those who had had more than 50% of the tumour removed and those who had had less than 50% of the tumour removed. In practical terms this usually meant that either the patient had had a very large proportion of tumour re-

Table 11. Results recorded in the levamisole trial in advanced ovarian cancer following surgical removal of only a small proportion of the tumor burden

Number	Complete response (%)	Partial response (%)	Drugs used
24	42	21	CYCLO + Depostat + placebo
25	48	20	CYCLO + Depostat + levamisole

Key: CYCLO, Cyclophosphamide; Depostat, gestronol hexanoate

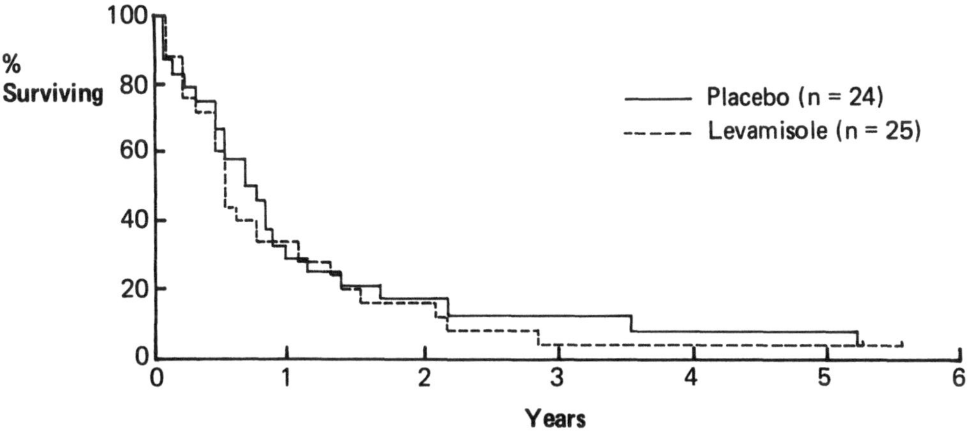

Fig. 6. Levamisole trial for advanced ovarian cancer: Survival of patients in whom the majority of tumour had not been removed and who received conventional chemotherapy with a combination of cyclophosphamide and gestronol hexanoate (Depostat), together with either levamisole or placebo on a randomized double-blind basis. The curves are not probability curves but represent actual survival

moved or had had little more than a biopsy. All patients received single-agent chemotherapy consisting of IV cyclophosphamide 200 mg daily for 5 days, followed by cyclophosphamide 50 mg PO four times a day continuously, the dose of cyclophosphamide being varied to maintain the patient's white cell count between 1.5 and $2.0 \times 10^9/1$. Patients also received gestronol hexanoate (Depostat) 200 mg IM once a week. This form of treatment has previously been shown to be reasonably effective and relatively non-toxic (Guthrie, 1979). In addition to cytotoxic treatment, patients were also randomized to receive either levamisole or placebo on a double-blind basis, the dose being one tablet three times a day for 3 consecutive days once a fortnight. Levamisole is an anthelmintic with the property of restoring cell-mediated immune response to normal, even in patients receiving cytotoxic chemotherapy. Treatment was started 7 days after laparotomy and was continued for as long as the patient was in remission or for 5 years, whichever was the shorter. The levamisole/placebo code was not broken until the death of the patient or at 5 years, whichever came earlier.

Table 12. Results recorded in the levamisole trial in advanced ovarian cancer following surgical removal of most of the tumour burden

Number	Complete response (%)	Partial response (%)	Drugs used
25	48	20	CYCLO + Depostat + placebo
25	68	4	CYCLO + Depostat + levamisole

Key: CYCLO, Cyclophosphamide; Depostat = gestronol hexanoate

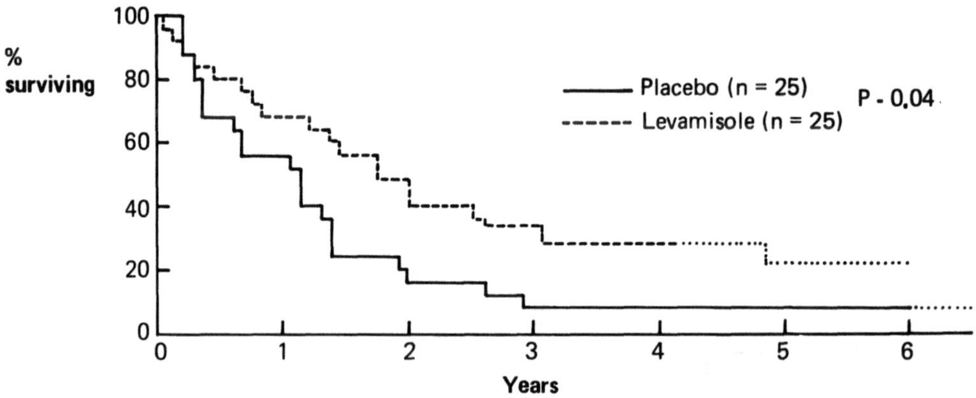

Fig. 7. Levamisole trial for advanced ovarian cancer: Survival of patients in whom the majority of tumour had been removed and who received conventional chemotherapy with a combination of cyclophosphamide and gestronol hexanoate (Depostat), together with either levamisole or placebo on a randomized double-blind basis. The curves represent actual survival until the fine dotted lines, at which time they become probability curves. The difference is statistically significant ($p = 0.04$, Mann Whitney U test)

The results recorded in patients in whom most of the tumour was not removed are shown in Table 11. There has been a non-significant increase in response rate with the use of levamisole, but as might be expected in patients with bulky disease, use of levamisole does not produce any increase in survival, as is shown in the survival curves depicted in Fig. 6. In the group in which most of the tumour was removed, the picture is different. Table 12 shows a much higher complete remission rate for those who received levamisole as opposed to placebo, and furthermore, this increase in complete remission is translated into greater survival, as shown in Fig. 7. The difference between these two curves is significant ($P = 0.04$. Mann-Whitney U test). If no further deaths occur in the levamisole-treated group within the next 11 months the 5-year survival rate for this group will be 24%, which compares well with the 8% 5-year survival rate for the placebo group. A detailed analysis of this trial will not take place until the remaining patients have survived to 5 years or died.

Conclusion

Assessment of the results of clinical trials with reference to remission alone is not always in the best interests of the patient, and the assessment should rather take account of length of survival coupled with quality of life. The hope raised by the increase in survival shown in the last two trials should encourage new endeavours directed at improvement of the results of treatment of this particular cancer. Some authors already claim that improvement, but unfortunately such claims do not stand up to close scrutiny. Perhaps the words of Claude Bernard (1878, English translation in 1949) are a fitting end to this chapter:

"It is what we think we know already that often prevents us from learning."

References

Alberts DS, Moon TE, Stephens RA, Wilson H, Oishi N, Hilgers RD, O'Toole R, Thigpen JT (1979) Randomized study of chemoimmunotherapy for advanced ovarian carcinoma: A preliminary report of a Southwest Oncology Group Study. Cancer Treat Rep 63: 325-331

Aure JC, Høeg K, Kolstad P (1971) Clinical and histologic studies of ovarian carcinoma. Long-term follow-up of 990 cases. Obstet Gynecol 37: 1-9

Barlow JJ, Blumenson LE (1979) Letter to the Editor. N Engl J Med 300: 676

Barlow JJ, Piver MS, Lele SB (1980) High-dose methotrexate with "RESCUE" plus cyclophosphamide as initial chemotherapy in ovarian adenocarcinoma. A randomized trial with observations on the influence of C. parvum immunotherapy. Cancer 46: 1333-1338

Bernard C (1878) An introduction to the study of experimental medicine. Schuman, New York, 1949

Bolis G, Bortolozzi G, Carinelli G, D'Incalci M, Gramellini F, Morasca L, Mangioni C (1980) Low-dose cyclophosphamide versus Adriamycin plus cyclophosphamide in advanced ovarian cancer. A randomized clinical study. Cancer Chemother Pharmacol 4: 129-132

Bruckner HW, Cohen CJ, Goldberg JD, Kabakow B, Wallach RC, Deppe G, Greenspan EM, Gusberg SB, Holland JF (1981) Improved chemotherapy for ovarian cancer with *cis*-diamminedichloroplatinum and Adriamycin. Cancer 47: 2288-2294

Bush RS (1979) Letter to the Editor. N Engl J Med 300: 676

Carmo-Pereira J, Costa FO, Henriques E, Ricardo JA (1981) Advanced ovarian carcinoma: A prospective and randomized clinical trial of cyclophosphamide versus combination cytotoxic chemotherapy (Hexa-CAF). Cancer 48: 1947-1951

Carmo-Pereira J, Costa FO, Henriques E (1982) *Cis*-platinum (P) Adriamycin (A) and hexamethylmelamine (H) vs cyclophosphamide (C) in advanced ovarian carcinoma - a randomized study. Proc ASCO 1: 107, C414

Decker DG, Fleming TR, Malkasian GD, Webb MJ, Jefferies JA, Edmonson JH (1982) Cyclophosphamide plus *cis*-platinum in combination: Treatment program for stage III or IV ovarian carcinoma. Obstet Gynecol 60: 481-487

Geisler HE, Minor JR, Eastlund ME (1976) The treatment of advanced ovarian carcinoma with high-dose intravenous cyclophosphamide. Gynecol Oncol 4: 43-52

Guthrie D (1979) The treatment of advanced cystadenocarcinoma of the ovary with gestronol and continuous oral cyclophosphamide. Br J Obstet Gynaecol 86: 497-500

Hudson CN (1980) Immunology and immunotherapy of ovarian cancer. In: Newman CE, Ford CHJ, Jordan JA (eds) Ovarian cancer. Pergamon, Oxford, pp 211-220

Izbicki RM, Baker LH, Samson MK, McDonald B, Vaitkevicius VK. (1977) 5-FU infusion and cyclophosphamide in the treatment of advanced ovarian cancer. Cancer Treat Rep 61: 1573-1575

Kessinger A, Foley JF, Lemon HM (1976) Quadrichemotherapy for advanced ovarian carcinoma. Obstet Gynecol 48: 134-136

Lloyd RE, Jones SE, Salmon SE, Durie BGM, McMahon LJ (1976) Combination chemotherapy with Adriamycin (NSC-123127) and cyclophosphamide (NSC-26271) for solid tumours: a phase II trial. Cancer Treat Rep 60: 77-83

Mangioni C, Bolis G, Natale N, Morasca L (1976) Continuous low-dose cyclophosphamide (NSC-26271) therapy in advanced ovarian cancer. Eur J Cancer 12: 353-356

Mangioni C, Bolis G, Valente I, Malina P, Sessa C (1981) *cis*-Diamminedichloroplatinum, Adriamycin, cyclophosphamide (PAC) vs hexamethylmelamine, Adriamycin and cyclophosphamide (HAC) in advanced ovarian cancer. Proc AACR/ASCO 22: 166, 660

Maskens AP, De Oliveira C, Dalesio O, di Re F, Lacave A, Namer M, Rotmensz N, Villani C, Wolff JP (1983) Effect of adding CDDP to the combination Adriamycin-cyclophosphamide in advanced ovarian cancer. In: Proceedings of the Second European Conference on Clinical Oncology and Cancer Nursing, Koningin Wilhelmina Fonds, Amsterdam, p 53

Medical Research Council's working party on ovarian cancer (1981) Medical Research Council study of chemotherapy in advanced ovarian cancer. Br J Obstet Gynaecol 88: 1174-1185

Miller AB, Klaassen DJ, Boyes DA, Dodds DJ, Gerulath A, Kirk ME, Levitt M, Pearson JG, Wall C (1980) Combination v. sequential therapy with melphalan, 5-fluorouracil and methotrexate for advanced ovarian cancer. Can Med Assoc J 123: 365-371

Neijt JP (1983) Combination chemotherapy in the treatment of advanced ovarian carcinoma. PhD thesis, University of Utrecht, The Netherlands, p 11

Neijt JP, Lindert ACM van, Vendrik CPJ, Roozendaal KJ, Struyvenberg A, Pinedo HM (1980) Treatment of advanced ovarian carcinoma with a combination of hexamethylmelamine, cyclophosphamide, methotrexate, and 5-fluorouracil (Hexa-CAF) in patients with and without previous treatment. Cancer Treat Rep 64: 323-326

Omura GA, Ehrlich CE, Blessing JA (1982) A randomized trial of cyclophosphamide (C) plus Adriamycin (A) with or without *cis*-platinum (P) in ovarian carcinoma. Proc ASCO 1: 104, C-403

Omura GA, Morrow CP, Blessing JA, Miller A, Buchsbaum HJ, Homesley HD, Leone L. (1983) A randomized comparison of melphalan versus melphalan plus hexamethylmelamine versus adriamycin plus cyclophosphamide in ovarian carcinoma. Cancer 51: 783-789

Park RC, Blom J, Disaia PJ, Lagasse LD, Blessing JA. (1980) Treatment of women with disseminated or recurrent advanced ovarian cancer with melphalan alone, in combination with 5-fluorouracil and dactinomycin, or with the combination of cytoxan, 5-flourouracil and dactinomycin. Cancer 45: 2529-2542

Parker LM, Griffiths CT, Yankee RA, Knapp RC, Canellos GP, Lokich JJ (1978) Adriamycin (A)/Cyclophosphamide (C) and surgical treatment of advanced ovarian cancer. AACR/ASCO 19: 399, C372

Parker LM, Griffiths CT, Yankee RA, Canellos GP, Gelman R, Knapp RC, Richman CM, Tobias JS, Weiner RS, Frei E (1980) Combination chemotherapy with Adriamycin-cyclophosphamide for advanced ovarian carcinoma. Cancer 46: 669-674

Piver MS, Barlow JJ, Yazigi R, Blumenson LE (1978) Melphalan chemotherapy in advanced ovarian carcinoma. Obstet Gynecol 51: 352-356

Schwartz PE, Lawrence R, Katz M (1981) Combination chemotherapy for advanced ovarian cancer: A prospective randomized trial comparing hexamethylmelamine and cyclophosphamide to doxorubicin and cyclophosphamide. Cancer Treat Rep 65: 137-141

Sturgeon JFG, Fine S, Gospodarowicz MK, Dembo AJ, Bean HA, Bush RS, Beale FA, Pringle JF, Thomas GM, Herman JG (1982) A randomized trial of melphalan alone versus combination chemotherapy in advanced ovarian cancer. Proc ASCO 1: 108, C418

Tobias JS, Griffiths CT (1976) Management of ovarian carcinoma. Current concepts and future prospects (Second of two parts.) N Engl J Med 294: 877-882

Tropé C. for the Swedish Cooperative Ovarian Cancer Study Group (1981) A prospective and randomized trial comparison of melphalan versus Adriamycin-melphalan in advanced ovarian carcinoma. Proc AACR/ASCO 22: 469, C533

Turbow MM, Jones H, Yu VK, Greenberg B, Hannigan J, Torti FM (1980) Chemotherapy of ovarian carcinoma: A comparison of melphalan versus Adriamycin-cyclophosphamide. Proc AACR/ASCO 21: 196, 785

Vogl SE, Kaplan B, Pagano M (1982) Diamminedichloroplatinum (D) - based combination chemotherapy (CT) is superior to melphalan (M) for advanced ovarian cancer (Ov Ca) when age is $\geqslant 50$ and tumour diameter > 2 cms. Proc ASCO 1: 119, C-462

Vogl SE, Pagano M, Kaplan BH, Greenwald E, Arseneau J, Bennett B (1983) cis-platin-based combination chemotherapy for advanced ovarian cancer. High overall response rate with curative potential only in women with small tumor burdens. Cancer 51: 2024-2030

Wagstaff J, Buckley H, Crowther D (1983) A trial of single-agent cyclophosphamide versus cisplatinum, bleomycin and cyclophosphamide combination in ovarian cancer. In: Proceedings of the of the Second European Conference on Clinical Oncology and Cancer Nursing, Koningin Wilhelmina Fonds, Amsterdam, p 46

Wilbur D, Rentschler R, Wagner R, Boice C, Keeney E, King A, and Hilliard D (1983) Randomized trial of the addition of cis-diamminodichloroplatinum (DDP) and/or BCG to cyclophosphamide (CTX) chemotherapy (chemo) for ovarian carcinoma. Proc ASCO 2: 147, C-574

Williams CJ, Mead GM, Green JA, Macbeth FR, Whitehouse JMA, Harvey VJ, Slevin ML, Shepherd J, Golding P (1983) A randomized study of cisplatin, Adriamycin and cyclophosphamide (PACe) versus chlorambucil (CB) in Stage III and IV ovarian carcinoma. Proc ASCO 2: 156, C-611

Young RC, Chabner BA, Hubbard SP, Fisher RI, Bender RA, Anderson T, Simon RM, Canellos GP, DeVita VT (1978) Advanced ovarian adenocarcinoma. A prospective clinical trial of melphalan (L-PAM) versus combination chemotherapy. N Engl J Med 299: 1261-1266

Chemotherapy for Malignant Ovarian Germ Cell Tumours

E. S. Newlands, R. H. J. Begent, G. J. S. Rustin, L. Holden, and
K. D. Bagshawe*

Department of Medical Oncology, Charing Cross Hospital, London W6 8RF, United Kingdom

Introduction

Although benign ovarian teratomas are relatively common and constitute approximately 20% of all ovarian tumours, malignant germ cell tumours are much less common and account for only about 1% (Fox and Langley 1976). In spite of their rarity, malignant ovarian germ cell tumours are important for two reasons: the first is that the average age at presentation is less than 20 years and, secondly, following recent improvements in their management it should now be rare for patients with these tumours to succumb from their disease. The pathology of malignant ovarian germ cell tumours is complex and most classifications are based upon modifications of the World Health Organisation (WHO) system of 1973 (e.g. Norris and Adam 1981). One practical simplification of the WHO classification is shown in Table 1. It is important that the histology is integrated with the additional information that is available from immunoperoxidase staining and the serum tumour markers human chorionic gonadotrophin (HCG), alphafetoprotein (AFP) and placental alka-

Table 1. Classification of malignant germ cell tumours of the ovary (Begent 1983)

A. Dysgerminoma
B. Endodermal sinus tumour
C. Teratomas
  1. Immature (malignant) teratoma
  2. Mature cystic teratoma with malignant transformation
  3. Monodermal or highly specialised
    a. Struma ovarii
    b. Carcinoid
    c. Strumal carcinoid
    d. Others
D. Embryonal carcinoma
E. Choriocarcinoma
F. Combination germ cell tumour

* We thank all the gynaecologists, surgeons and radiotherapists who referred patients to us, and the staff at the Charing Cross Hospital for excellent support. The initial supply of cis-platinum was from the NCI, Bethesda, Md., and the initial supply of etoposide was from Bristol-Myers Co. Ltd. We thank the Cancer Research Campaign for support of two of the authors (R. H. J. B. and G. J. S. R.), the Medical Research Council for support of studies on tumour markers and Lederle Laboratories for support for the data analysis

Ovarian Cancer, Ed. by N. M. Bleehen

line phosphatase (PLAP). When all these three techniques are taken into account, the incidence of combination germ cell tumours is more common than had been previously recognised. While the pathology of the various types of malignant ovarian germ cell tumours is complex, as will be discussed later, the clinical management has become simpler.

Integral to the management of malignant ovarian germ cell tumours is routine and regular monitoring of the serum tumour markers. The majority of malignant ovarian germ cell tumours produce at least one of the following markers: HCG, AFP, PLAP and lactate dehydrogenase (LDH). This last one is a less specific marker but can be useful. In many cases, serial tumour marker estimations provide the most accurate monitor of progression or regression of a germ cell tumour. It is now recognised that the initial serum concentration of HCG and/or AFP is one of the most important prognostic variables affecting the clinical outcome in male patients with metastatic germ cell tumours (Germa-Lluch et al. 1980; Newlands et al. 1983).

Management and Staging Procedures

Although malignant ovarian germ cell tumours are rare, it is important for any surgeon operating on a young woman (particularly under the age of 20) with a pelvic mass to be aware that advances in management have made radical surgery less necessary. While as much tumour should be removed as possible, the aim should be to preserve the opposite ovary and uterus. Following the histological diagnosis, the main staging procedures include twice-weekly serum samples for the tumour markers specified above and thoracic and abdominal computerised tomography (CT). CT scanning provides the most accurate method currently available for detecting pulmonary metastases and is useful in detecting para-aortic node involvement, liver metastases and pelvic masses. However, the transcoelomic spread that is common in malignant ovarian germ cell tumours is not easily detected with this technique. In selected patients, lymphangiography may be indicated if the CT scan is normal, since this technique can detect intranodal metastases below the resolution of CT scanning. Ultrasound is useful for detecting hepatic and pelvic disease and can also be helpful in monitoring para-aortic nodes.

Following these investigations, patients are classified according to the International Federation of Gynaecology and Obstetrics (FIGO) staging for ovarian tumours. In most centres the management of the patient will depend on whether or not the histology and serum markers (i.e. normal HCG and AFP) indicate a pure dysgerminoma or one of the other cell types of malignant germ cell tumour. Dysgerminomas are highly radiosensitive, and radiotherapy has been considered the standard post-operative treatment for patients with this tumour. The possibility of preserving fertility by limited-field irradiation of the pelvis may be practicable in selected patients and is discussed more fully in Bagshawe et al. (1983). In our experience dysgerminomas are highly sensitive to chemotherapy and this alternative should be carefully considered in those patients in whom preservation of fertility is possible. In patients with other cell types of malignant germ cell tumour (see Table 1) those with metastatic disease should now be treated with combination chemotherapy and this will be discussed later. However, given the much greater efficacy of current therapy for eliminating metastatic disease, those patients who are stage I on all staging investigations discussed above do not need to receive routine adjuvant chemotherapy. For several years our policy has been to watch these patients closely with serial serum tumour marker estimations and close clinical and radiological follow-up. Our experience in both the germ cell tumours of the ovary and their male counterpart in the testis is that all patients managed in this way can be salvaged with chemotherapy if the metastatic disease is detected at an early stage. This approach allows the majority of patients with stage I disease to receive no additional treatment after their initial surgery.

Chemotherapy

It has been recognised since 1960 that malignant germ cell tumours can respond dramatically to cytotoxic chemotherapy. However, until the middle of the 1970s the majority of patients who responded initially to cytotoxic chemotherapy subsequently developed drug-resistant disease and died. Our experience at Charing Cross Hospital during this period was similar and, using drug combinations including methotrexate, actinomycin D, cyclophosphamide, vinblastine, bleomycin and mithramcyin, we had three long-term survivors (at 9+, 13+ and 15+ years) out of 12 patients treated during this period. One of the most widely used drug combinations of the 1970s was vincristine, actinomycin D and cyclophosphamide (VAC). Slayton et al. (1978) reported 39 patients treated with this combination and, although 16 out of 23 patients with stage I and II A disease survived, only 8 out of 16 with stages II B–IV survived. Cangir et al. (1978) reported that 8 out of 8 patients with stage I and II disease survived although in the group with stage IV disease only 1 out of 5 patients survived. It appears from the reported series using VAC chemotherapy that this approach is able to control small volumes of tumour but that results with large-volume metastases are poor. In most of these series VAC chemotherapy is continued for up to 2 years and it is now clearly recognised that chemotherapy of this duration which includes an alkylating agent carries a risk of inducing second tumours (Greene et al. 1982).

In the middle 1970s two new highly active cytotoxic drugs, cis-platinum and etoposide (VP 16-213), were introduced into the management of malignant germ cell tumours. Several groups have reported results using a combination of cis-platinum, vinblastine and bleomycin (PVB). Williams et al. (1981) reported a series of 30 patients of whom 24 were evaluable and 13 (54%) were in complete remission at this time. They concluded that the prognosis was related to the residual tumour volume following surgery but not the histological type of germ cell tumour. Carlson et al. (1983), also using PVB, reported 9 survivors out of 9 patients, although the majority of their patients had stage I disease. Wiltshaw et al. (1982) treated 8 patients with endodermal sinus (yolk sac) tumour with PVB and obtained 7 out of 8 complete remissions. Using drug combinations with vinblastine, actinomycin D, bleomycin and cis-platinum, Bradof et al. (1982) reported 17 patients but only 9 of these were alive and one had persisting disease. One reason for these relatively poor results may be the extensive prior treatment that many of their patients had received.

At the Charing Cross Hospital we have pioneered a different approach to the chemotherapy of metastatic germ cell tumours. Shortly after the introduction of cis-platinum we identified the significant activity of etoposide (VP 16-213) against malignant germ cell tumours (Newlands and Bagshawe 1977). We have integrated both these drugs into sequential chemotherapy (POMB/ACE) and, using these regimens, have experience in treating over 170 patients with malignant germ cell tumours between 1977 and 1984. While the majority of these patients are male, we have managed patients of both sexes in the same way, and as far as we can tell there are no major biological differences between the germ cell tumours occurring in either sex. The chemotherapy schedules that we use are shown in Table 2. Patients initially receive two courses of POMB followed by ACE. Subsequently

Table 2. POMB/ACE sequential chemotherapy

POMB

Day 1: Vincristine 1 mg/m^2 intravenously (i. v.), methotrexate 100 mg/m^2 i. v., followed by methotrexate 200 mg/m^2 as a 12 h infusion

Day 2: Bleomycin 15 mg given as a 24 h infusion, folinic acid rescue 24 h after the start of the methotrexate in a dose of 15 mg 12-hourly for 4 doses

Day 3: Bleomycin infusion 15 mg by 24 h infusion

Day 4: Forced diuresis with mannitol and hydration at the rate of 1 l/h for 3 h before cis-platinum 120 mg/m^2 as a short i. v. infusion, and diuresis with mannitol at 1 l/h for a further 3 h. Hydration until the patient stops vomiting. Since 1981 patients have routinely received 3 g magnesium sulphate i. v. as part of the hydration schedule before administration of the cis-platinum

ACE

Etoposide 100 mg/m^2 i. v., days 1-5; actinomycin D 0.5 mg i. v., days 3, 4 and 5; cyclophosphamide 500 mg/m^2 i. v. day 5

OMB

As for POMB, omitting day 4 (hydration and cis-platinum)

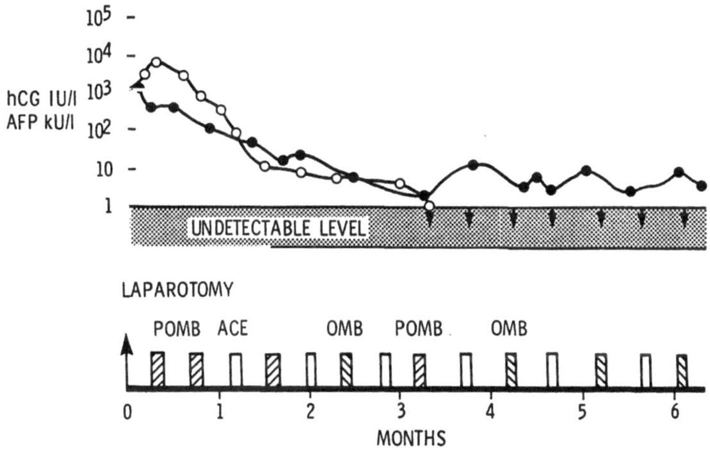

Fig. 1. Tumour marker response in a patient with stage IV combined germ cell tumour, illustrating the pattern and duration of sequential combination chemotherapy. In patients receiving multiple courses of cis-platinum therapy the AFP concentrations can remain above the normal baseline and present problems of interpretation (Coppack et al. 1983). This patient remains in complete remission and off all treatment.
Drugs: cis-platinum (P); vincristine (O); methotrexate (M); bleomycin (B); actinomycin D (A); cyclophosphamide (C); etoposide (E)

POMB is alternated with ACE until patients are in biochemical remission as measured by hCG, AFP, PLAP and LDH values. The usual number of courses of POMB required is three to five. Patients then continue alternating ACE with OMB until biochemical remission has been sustained for approximately 12 weeks. The sequence of treatment schedules is shown in Fig. 1. The duration of treatment has been adjusted to the requirements of the individual patient and no maintenance therapy has been given. At the end of chemotherapy, patients have been re-staged by thoracic and abdominal CT scans and residual masses have been resected where this has been feasible. Using this approach, and with

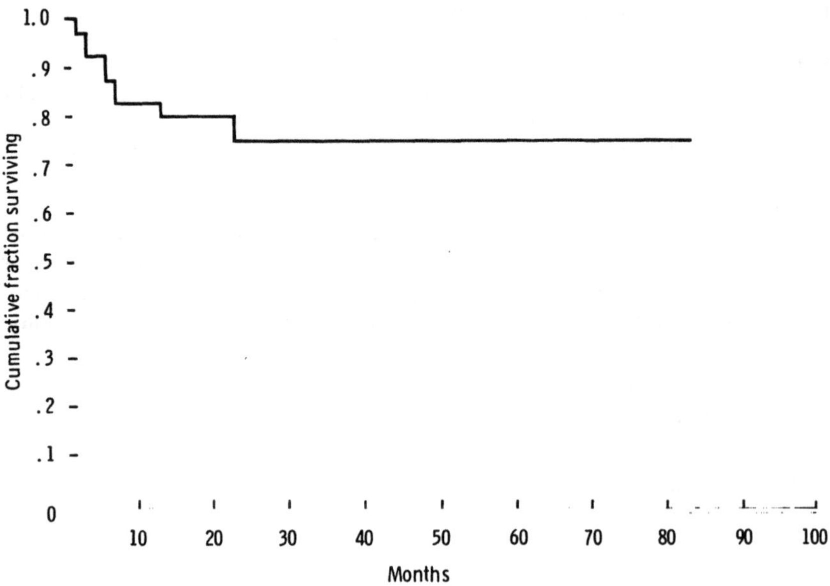

Fig. 2. Overall survival of 31 patients with malignant ovarian germ cell tumours

suitable modification for patients with brain metastases, the majority of patients even with very large-volume metastatic disease can achieve complete remissions (Newlands et al. 1983).

We previously reported our initial experience up to 1981 using POMB/ACE chemotherapy in ovarian germ cell tumours (Newlands et al. 1982). Since that report we now have 31 female patients with malignant germ cell tumours who have completed treatment to 1 January 1984. We have repeated the multivariate analysis that we performed in the male patients and, although the series for the female patients is relatively small, the pattern of survival is very similar. When analysed by stage, unlike other series, there is no significant difference between groups. For stage IM (biochemical evidence of metastatic disease only) 4 out of 4 patients are alive; for stage II, 7 out of 10 patients are alive; for stage III, 6 out of 8 patients are alive, and for stage IV, 7 out of 9 patients are alive. Four out of 6 patients with widespread liver metastases are alive in remission.

The overall survival by life table analysis of patients who have completed treatment is shown in Fig. 2. This projects a survival of 75%. When separated by histology, all 4 patients with metastatic or recurrent dysgerminomas are in remission, indicating the extreme chemosensitivity of this tumour to POMB/ACE chemotherapy. There was no difference in survival between patients with different tumour histologies. Thus for endodermal sinus tumour survival was 7 out of 9 (78%); for choriocarcinoma, 2 out of 2 (100%); and for the combination germ cell tumours, 12 out of 16 (75%). In analysing patients with the various types of malignant ovarian teratoma by the production of the tumour markers HCG and AFP, there is a trend towards a poorer prognosis in patients with high HCG (> 50000 IU/l) and/or AFP (> 500 kU/l) at the time of starting treatment (Fig. 3). In the larger series of male patients the initial serum concentration of HCG and/or AFP is one of the most important prognostic variables (Newlands et al. 1983).

In this group of malignant ovarian teratomas the most important initial prognostic variable was prior treatment with radiotherapy and/or chemotherapy (Fig. 4). Only 2 out

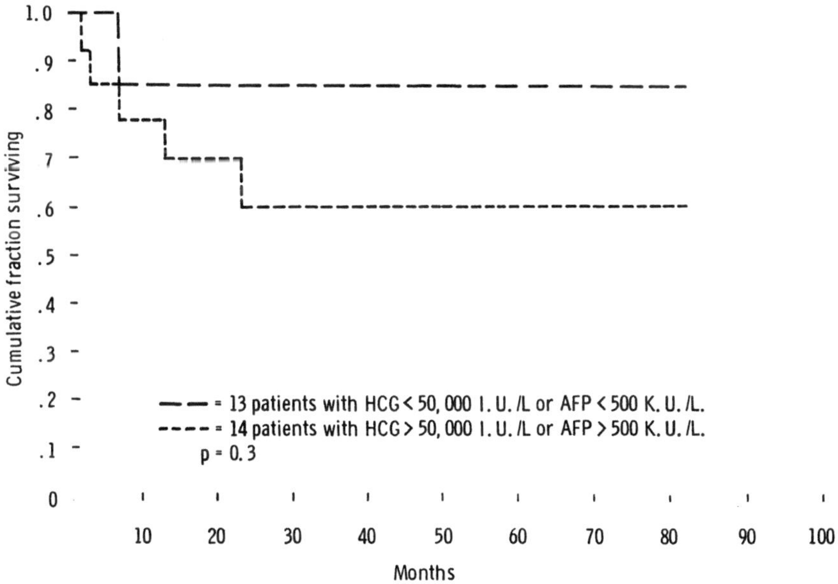

Fig. 3. Analysis of patients with malignant ovarian teratomas by the initial serum concentrations of HCG and AFP

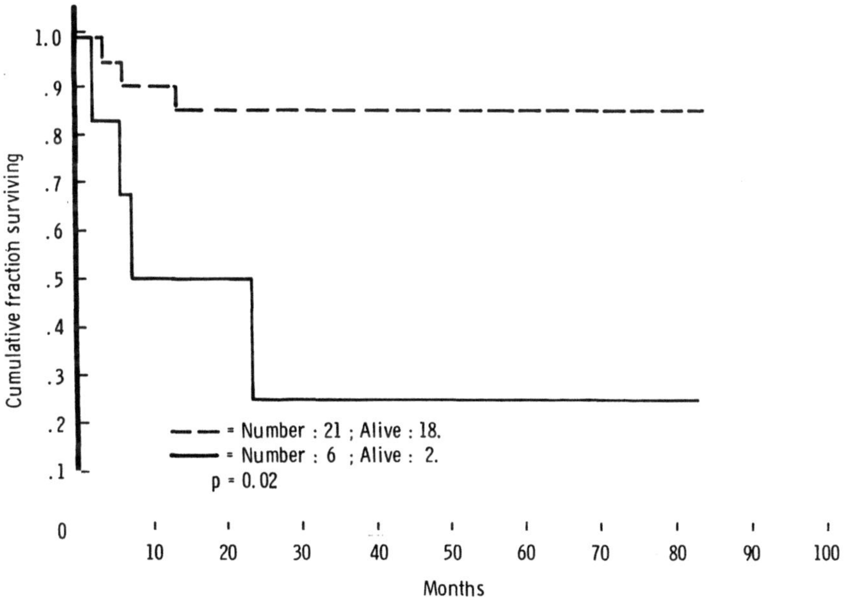

Fig. 4. Analysis of patients with malignant ovarian teratomas by prior radiotherapy and/or chemotherapy. The continuous and dashed lines represent groups of patients who had or had not received prior radiotherapy and/or chemotherapy respectively

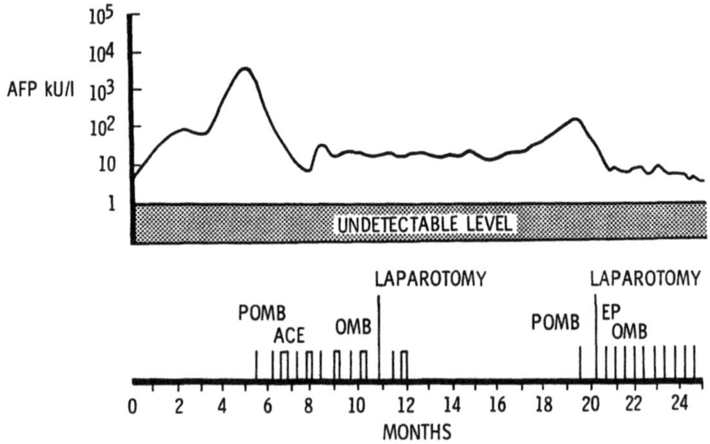

Fig. 5. Patient who relapsed following VAC chemotherapy. After treatment with POMB/ACE the AFP remained above the normal baseline but at a concentration which is not diagnostic of residual tumour (Coppack et al. 1983). For further details of her management, see text

of 6 patients with prior radiotherapy and/or chemotherapy obtained a complete remission, in contrast to 84% of 21 patients who had received no prior treatment apart from surgery. With a maximum follow-up time of 82 months, this clearly indicates that few patients with metastatic ovarian germ cell tumours should die from their disease provided that they are treated appropriately in a specialist centre from the outset.

We have tried a variety of modifications of POMB/ACE chemotherapy in patients who have been referred after failing on alternative chemotherapy, including both VAC and PVB. The problem here has not been in getting an initial anti-tumour response but in obtaining stable complete remissions. This is illustrated in Fig. 5. Although the patient responded clinically and biochemically (AFP) to POMB/ACE chemotherapy and had no evidence of disease at laparotomy, the tumour relapsed again after an interval of 7 months. On this occasion the site of relapse was identified by radioimmunolocalisation with iodinated anti-AFP and this was resected. In order to reduce toxicity, the chemotherapy we are currently using in this context is etoposide (200 mg/m^2) combined with cisplatinum (100 mg/m^2 by 24-h infusion) alternating with OMB. This patient currently remains in remission.

At present there is no evidence of long-term side-effects using POMB/ACE chemotherapy in these patients. The children treated are developing normally and some of them have gone through puberty without any evidence of endocrine dysfunction. These patients are menstruating normally and the first of them is pregnant, confirming that fertility in the female as well as the male can be preserved following POMB/ACE chemotherapy. Cytotoxic chemotherapy given by intermittent schedules over a limited period does not necessarily have a major long-term effect on ovarian function, as is shown in our results in patients with gestational choriocarcinoma. In this series of 445 patients, 86% succeeded in having at least one live birth (Rustin et al. 1984). We hope that our patients with germ cell tumours will be as productive.

References

Bagshawe KD, Begent RHJ, Glaser M, House M, Newlands ES (1983) The Ovary. In: KD Bagshawe, ES Newlands, RHJ Begent (eds) Germ Cell Tumours. WB Saunders, London, pp 215-232

Begent RHJ (1983) Germ Cell Tumours. In J Studd (ed) Progress in Obstetrics and Gynaecology, vol 3. Churchill Livingstone, Edinburgh, pp 174-186

Bradof JE, Hakes TB, Ochoa M, Golbey R (1982) Germ Cell Malignancies of the Ovary. Cancer 50: 1070-1075

Cangir A, Smith J, Van Eys J (1978) Improved prognosis in children with ovarian cancers following modified VAC (vincristine sulphate, dactinomycin and cyclophosphamide) chemotherapy. Cancer 42: 1234-1238

Carlson RW, Sikic BI, Turbow MM, Ballon SC (1983) Combination cisplatin, vinblastine and bleomycin chemotherapy (PVB) for malignant germ cell tumours of the ovary. J Clin Oncol 1: 645-651

Coppack S, Newlands ES, Dent J, Mitchell H, Goka G, Bagshawe KD (1983) Problems of interpretation of serum concentrations of alpha-foetoprotein (AFP) in patients receiving cytotoxic chemotherapy for malignant germ cell tumours. Br J Cancer 48: 335-340

Fox H, Langley FA (1976) Germ cell tumours with predominantly embryonic development. In: H Fox, FA Langley (eds) Tumours of the ovary. Heinemann, London, pp 210-230

Germa-Lluch JR, Begent RHJ, Bagshawe KD (1980) Tumour marker levels and prognosis in malignant teratomas of the testis. Br J Cancer 42: 850-855

Greene MH, Boice JD, Greer BE, Blessing JA, Dembo AJ (1982) Acute non-lymphocytic leukaemia after therapy with alkylating agents for ovarian carcinoma. N Engl J Med 307: 1416-1421

Newlands ES, Bagshawe KD (1977) Epipodophyllin derivative (VP 16213) in malignant teratomas and choriocarcinomas. Lancet II: 87

Newlands ES, Begent RHJ, Rustin GJS, Bagshawe KD (1982) Potential for cure in metastatic ovarian teratomas and dysgerminomas. Br J Obstet Gynaecol 89: 555-560

Newlands ES, Begent RHJ, Rustin GJS, Parker D, Bagshawe KD (1983) Further advances in the management of malignant teratomas of the testis and other sites. Lancet 1: 948-951

Norris HJ, Adam AE (1981) Malignant germ cell tumours of the ovary. In: M Coppleson (ed) Gynaecologic Oncology. Churchill Livingstone, Edinburgh, pp 680-696

Rustin GJS, Booth M, Dent J, Salt S, Rustin F, Bagshawe KD (1984) Pregnancy after cytotoxic chemotherapy for gestational trophoblastic tumours. Br Med J 288: 103-106

Slayton RE, Hreshchyshyn MM, Silverberg SG, Shingleton HM, Park RC, Disaia PJ, Blessing JA (1978) Treatment of malignant ovarian germ cell tumours. Cancer 42: 390-398

Williams S, Slayton R, Silverberg S, Ehrlich C, Einhorn L, Blessing J (1981) Response of malignant ovarian germ cell tumours to cis-platinum, vinblastine and bleomycin (PVB). Proc Am Soc Clin Oncol Abstr C-509

Wiltshaw E, Stuart-Harris R, Barker GH, Gowing NFC, Raju S (1982) Chemotherapy of endodermal sinus tumour (yolk sac tumour) of the ovary: Preliminary communication. J R Soc Med 75: 888-892

Subject Index

MIX
Papier aus verantwortungsvollen Quellen
Paper from responsible sources
FSC® C105338

If you have any concerns about our products,
you can contact us on
ProductSafety@springernature.com

In case Publisher is established outside the EU,
the EU authorized representative is:
Springer Nature Customer Service Center GmbH
Europaplatz 3, 69115 Heidelberg, Germany

Printed by Libri Plureos GmbH
in Hamburg, Germany